MINDSET PREPARATION MOTIVATION

# CHAMPION
# MINDED

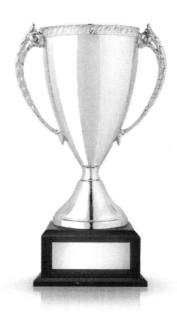

*Achieving Excellence in Sports and Life*

by **ALLISTAIR McCAW & JENNY W. ROBB**

# CHAMPION MINDED
*– Achieving Excellence in Sports and Life*
Copyright © 2017 Allistair McCaw

First Edition – August 2017

ISBN: 978-0-692-79154-7

Library of Congress Cataloging-in-Publication Data

Category: Athletic Coaching, Mindset, Motivational

Written by: Allistair McCaw | McCawMethod@gmail.com

Co-Authored & Edited by: Jenny W. Robb

Cover Design, Text Layout by: Eli Blyden | www.EliTheBookGuy.com

Printed in the United States of America by: A&A Printing | www.PrintShopCentral.com

ACT
LIVE
LOOK
THINK
PREPARE
COMMIT
COMPETE
COMMUNICATE

CHAMPION MINDED

# Disclaimer

# Table of Contents

MINDSET  PREPARATION  MOTIVATION

# CHAMPION
# MINDED

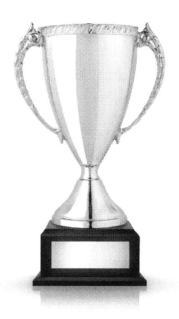

*Achieving Excellence in Sports and Life*

by **ALLISTAIR McCAW & JENNY W. ROBB**

# Introduction

## *Success Starts With Having A Vision.*

I believe all great accomplishments and achievements start with a vision. Many years ago, I had a vision for the front cover of my book. It included gold (the color that symbolizes a champion) and a shiny gold trophy. Like an athlete who has a vision of winning major championships, I had already seen the result in my mind a thousand times.

Champion Minded is written and designed to be a uniquely personal coach to athletes, an in-depth resource tool for coaches, and an insightful guide for parents. Each section progresses to the next level of training for preparation, mindset, and motivation: Preparing to Train, Learning to Train, Developmental Training, Competitive Training, Before Competition, During Competition, and After Competition. Each entry is written in the language of athletes with clear and to-the-point main ideas. Each section addresses physical, mental, and emotional areas to help athletes achieve their goals in sport and in life.

It is my hope that coaches and parents will use this book as a tool to help and to support their athletes. In each session I have with an athlete, I dedicate five minutes to a mindset message. With that in mind, this book provides a perfect resource for coaches to use with athletes.

Sport gives us so much. It teaches us about accountability, commitment, confidence, courage, discipline, gratitude, failure, values, humility, resilience and so much more. It reminds us how setting personal standards, committing to daily habits, and maintaining a positive perspective separates the good from the great. My goal for this book is to give back to sport, in the hope that these pages inspire you, guide you, and motivate you to train your mind and body for excellence in sport and in life.

A few years ago, I had an unforgettable conversation with Rory McIlroy, the #1 golfer in the world at the time. We were sitting on the plush, white couches in the players' lounge during the Rome Masters tennis tournament, both sipping a fine Italian coffee and sharing our experiences growing up in Northern Ireland. Rory grew up in Holywood, a small town not far from where my grandmother sometimes worked in a cafeteria. I was born in Belfast. As I frequently do when I meet athletes at the peak of their sport, I asked what he felt the key was to being a champion. Rory leaned back into the couch, paused and thought for a moment before replying, "a champion has to have a mind that is all about self-belief. It's all about how you feel about yourself and your game at that present time." In the fast-paced, competitive world of sports, something so simple is often incredibly difficult to grasp.

Upon saying our farewells, I remember walking down under to the players' locker rooms of the Foro Italico stadium and thinking to myself, "That's it! That is what I'm going to name my next book - *Champion Minded*." On that particular day, I decided to write this book.

A few weeks later, in Madrid, Spain, I met with Real Madrid soccer superstar, Ronaldo. During my very brief chat with the icon, I couldn't help but ask him the same question I'd asked Rory weeks earlier, "What makes a champion athlete?" His reply was pretty much the same as Rory, "Hard work, a mind of a champion, and a strong belief in yourself that you can do it."

## My Purpose and WHY

I wanted to write a book that athletes and coaches could really relate to. I am not a psychologist. I don't have a PhD. However, I do have the advantage of being a former professional athlete and now a coach of twenty-five years. In other wo'rds, I've been in the trenches fighting as an athlete and now I stand alongside them as they pursue greatness. As a coach to many athletes, including Olympians and world-class performers, I have seen what works and what doesn't. I've learned why some succeed and why some don't.

I wanted to write a book that was easy to read and easy to put into practice. In my line of work consulting with athletes, coaches and parents, I am often asked to refer a book on mindset or motivation. Even though there are many books out there, most are difficult for young athletes to read and to put into practice. They are written by incredibly intellectual people - psychologists and scientists - who I feel at times, struggle to bring across a message in "our language." My aim was to write a book that fused the way athletes best receive and learn information today - in short bursts. The goal was to keep the chapters short (1-2 pages), so that the message would stick.

One can easily apply this book's lessons and nuggets of advice to life as well as to sport. One of my driving purposes of this book was to bring the message across - if you are prepared to dedicate yourself and to work for it, you can achieve almost anything you want in life. Like Rory and Cristiano, if you believe in yourself and you are prepared to outwork the rest, great things can happen. If you apply yourself fully each day and aim to think, act, compete, look, prepare, communicate, commit, and live like a champion minded human being, greatness is possible. In fact, the eight elements I have just listed are what being champion minded is all about. It takes more than just an idea or dream to win. To be a champion in sport and in life requires your heart, mind, and soul.

You are not born mindset tough. You choose to be. Getting mindset tough means enduring experiences in your life. From those experiences, champion minded athletes and people develop grit. What is grit you ask? It's the ability to overcome challenges and to endure hardship. It's about handling and overcoming failure, and it's about getting up one more time after being knocked down.

A champion mindset is not about being gifted or talented. It's about being prepared, focused, disciplined, and having a deep unshakable belief in oneself. The reality is, some days you will feel great and some days you will feel terrible. Some days you are inspired and some days you can't even find the motivation to get out of bed. But here's what really matters: you have a vision and you believe in yourself, because there's no limit to what you can achieve. Your vision will drive you. Your job is to create a vision that makes you want to leap out of bed each morning and to attack the day.

My wish is that you use the lessons, encounters, experiences, and information I've compiled in this book to help you achieve and realize your greatest achievements. Believe that greatness is waiting for you. Don't wait for it. Step forward into it. Becoming champion minded is not a sacrifice, it is a choice, you were destined for greatness, not just in a sport, but in life too.

Lastly, I have always believed that even if you get just one thing from a book that can help you on your journey, then it's been worthwhile. So with that in mind, it's time to grab that bright yellow highlighter and become champion minded.

- Allistair McCaw, August 2017

# Being Champion Minded

## *A Champion Minded Athlete Is...*

**Accountable:** They take responsibility for their own actions.

**Coachable:** They listen and welcome feedback.

**Competitive:** They love the challenge and embrace the struggle.

**Confident:** They believe in themselves.

**Consistent:** They commit to daily habits, behaviors, and actions.

**Courageous:** They are willing to take risks.

**Determined:** They are eager and prepared to go the extra mile.

**Disciplined:** They have self-control.

**Driven:** They wake up each day with a desire to be better than the day before.

**Focused:** They eliminate distractions.

**Grateful:** They understand that playing sport is a privilege.

**Hard Working:** They commit to giving extra effort.

**Optimistic:** They believe that they can and will succeed.

**Organized:** They thrive with structure and routine.

**Positive:** They are able to adapt in challenging circumstances rather than making excuses.

**Prepared:** They are meticulous in their preparation, knowing it is the root of confidence.

**Process Minded:** They stay in the moment, focusing on performance first, before results.

**Resilient:** They are able to bounce back from setbacks quickly.

**Respectful:** They respect their opponents but never fear them.

**Self-Motivated:** They have an inner drive and strong purpose.

M

*Becoming champion minded doesn't only happen on the court, field, or in the gym.  It starts with having a vision, and then adhering to the habits, routines, and standards of a champion.*

*Becoming champion minded involves acting, living, looking, thinking, preparing, committing, competing, and communicating like a champion.*

# SECTION 1:

# *Preparing to Train*

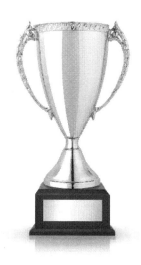

# Become Your Vision

*Before the goal is set,
the vision must be clear.*

A vision is a conscious decision and an image of where you see yourself in the future. Different from a dream, a vision is something more tangible. Whereas a dream is a more abstract idea, vague and elusive, you can nearly *grasp* a vision. A dream can exist subtly and undefined. A vision has a clear purpose and leads to a plan of action.

In an interview during the Rio Olympics with swimmer Michael Phelps, the most decorated Olympian of all time, he spoke about the vision he had as a young boy growing up in Baltimore, "I can remember sitting in the classroom at school envisioning myself winning a gold medal at the Olympics. Little did I know that that vision would lead to a few more medals! In fact, I still do visualize my races and have seen myself going fast."

In a television interview when he was ten years old, Novak Djokovic said he saw himself being a professional player and winning grand slam tournaments! Arrogance? No. Young Novak already possessed a self-belief and a vision for his future. He went on to be ranked number one in the world and to win numerous grand slam titles, including a career grand slam.

I remember drawing a picture as a young kid with the words: "Allistair McCaw – World Champion." Back then, my vision was to become a world champion in the sport of Duathlon (bike-run). Stuck above my bed for me to see every morning on waking and every night before sleeping, that picture motivated me to action. Even though I never reached my goal, I did go on to race professionally and to compete in five world championships! Today, as a coach and mentor, I ask my athletes to write down their vision and goals. To get somewhere, you first need to know where you want to go. It all starts with your vision. Your vision will provide the road map on the journey to achieving success and greatness. Having a vision gives purpose to your daily routines and your personal standards. The champion minded athlete understands that all greatness starts with a vision.

\* \* \*

*"If you are working on something that you really care about, you don't have to be pushed. The vision pulls you."*

- Steve Jobs

*Motivation doesn't come from passion.*
*It comes from having a vision*
*and purpose.*

# Setting Your Standards

*Your standards are reflected in
what you consistently do.*

Athletes: your standards are how you hold yourself accountable. Standards represent the things you choose as acceptable behaviors and practices based on your personal expectations. Your core values and the beliefs, which influence your behavior, form your standards. Champion minded athletes consistently adhere to incredibly high standards.

Recently, while speaking with Patrick Mourataglou, long-time coach of Serena Williams, he spoke about the strict standards that Serena expected of herself and her team, with the demands increasing each year. Even after two decades of great success on the women's professional tennis tour, she continually increases her standards.

Kobe Bryant is also well-known for his rigorous work ethic and his meticulously high standards. In a conversation with Tim DiFrancesco, LA Lakers' head strength and conditioning coach, he described Kobe saying, "His standards were so high that it was sometimes tough for some of the younger, newer guys to get to grips with it." Bryant entered the NBA directly after high school and won five NBA championships with the Lakers. He is an 18-time all-star, 15-time member of the All-NBA team, and 12-time member of the All-Defensive team. His four All-Star MVP awards are tied for the most in NBA history. At the 2008 and 2012 Summer olympics, he won gold medals as a member of team U.S.A. His statement,

"Everything negative - pressure, challenges - is an opportunity for me to rise," exemplifies his standards.

Maintaining high standards on a consistent basis will ultimately lead to greater results. Champion minded athletes hold themselves accountable to increasingly higher standards. They commit to a lifestyle that does not accept excuses or mediocrity. They are relentless in the pursuit of their goals.

Athletes: What are your standards? How would you rate your work ethic, attitude, and effort? Do your standards change when no one is watching? Do your standards reflect your goals? If you're not sure how to answer these questions, take a moment to sit down and write. Take time to reflect and to access yourself - what you are doing and why are you doing it? Are there areas in which you can raise your standards to meet your goals?*

\* \* \*

*Champion minded athletes
commit to higher standards.*

# 7 Habits of a Champion Minded Athlete

## *Are your habits helping you succeed?*

1.  A champion minded athlete accepts that they are not going to perform to their greatest expectations or at their highest level every time they compete. They still compete with a great attitude and give their best effort.

2.  A champion minded athlete understands that success does not lie in a one-off win or an occasional brilliant moment. Consistent performance at a high level leads to success.

3.  A champion minded athlete gives their best effort, bolstered by self-belief, even on the bad days. When performing at a sub-par level, champion minded athletes do not abandon hope of winning or slack off in their effort to find a way to win.

4.  A champion minded athlete does not compare their journey to anyone else's journey. They focus on the process and they are diligent in their daily routines.

5.  A champion minded athlete rises above obstacles. They are resilient and resourceful in the face of adversity. Rather than making excuses, they use their energy to find solutions.

6.  A champion minded athlete controls the controllables. They are not derailed by circumstances out of their control such as an opponent's bad behavior, an official's bad call, a spectator's bad etiquette, a teammate's poor performance, or changes in weather.

7. A champion minded athlete knows that not all wins are going to be pretty, but they are willing to win ugly. They don't give up just because they are having a bad day.

\* \* \*

*The biggest barrier to our own success is often ourselves.*

# A is for Attitude

*Your journey starts with your attitude.*

This is where it all begins. As the alphabet starts with the letter "A," so too does your journey to achieving success as an athlete and person. It all starts with the attitude you choose!

When it comes to sport, attitude is defined as your mindset in approaching, preparing for, and performing during practice and competition. Attitude is a way of thinking, which is reflected in your behaviors.

During my 25 years of coaching and consulting, I have observed many talented athletes and players whose careers never reached their full potential. Due to an attitude and a mindset which impeded their progress rather than nurturing their success, they failed.

Having spent time around world-class athletes and Olympians, I have come to realize it's easy to be good on the good days, but, when things aren't going according to plan, the great ones still rise to the top. Put simply, no matter the circumstances, it comes down to your attitude. A bad attitude is like having a flat tire - you're not going to get very far.

A champion minded athlete has a positive attitude and a forward-thinking mindset. They understand they can't always perform at their best level, but they know that by keeping a winning mindset and great attitude, they improve their chances for success.

The big difference between the champions and all other contenders, is that the champions are willing to work on building and developing their mindset everyday.

We only need to look to the Lebrons, Ronaldos, and Rafael Nadals of the world to see that champion athletes possess the traits and qualities to overcome adversity and to achieve greatness. These champion minded performers understand that it all starts with your attitude.

* * *

*The difference between failing and succeeding all comes down to the attitude you choose.*

# 10 Things to Expect on Your Athletic Journey

*Champion minded athletes know that success is a journey.*

1. **You will experience many highs and lows along the way.** These lines from Rudyard Kipling's *If* are emblazoned over the player's entrance to Wimbledon's Centre Court, "If you can meet with Triumph and Disaster/And treat those two imposters just the same."

2. **You will play your best and still lose.** Legendary coach John Wooden had a simple measure of success - peace of mind. According to Wooden, "Success is peace of mind which is a direct result of self-satisfaction in knowing you did your best to become the best that you are capable of becoming."

3. **You will lose some "friends" along the way.** American former professional baseball shortstop, Derek Jeter, who played 20 seasons in Major League Baseball for the New York Yankees, said, "Surround yourself with good people. People who are going to be honest with you and look out for your best interests."

4. **You will be misunderstood for your discipline and choice of lifestyle.** Retired Brazilian professional footballer, Pelé, widely regarded as the greatest football player of all time, said, "Success is no accident. It is hard work, perseverance, learning, studying, sacrifice, and most of all, love of what you are doing or learning to do."

5. **You will miss out on social events and family functions.** Pat Riley, American professional basketball executive, former coach and player in the NBA, said, "There are only two options regarding commitment. You're either IN or you're OUT. There's no such thing as life in-between."

6. **You will be sore - there will be pain.** Muhammad Ali, American professional boxer and one of the most significant and celebrated sports figures of the 20th century, famously said, "I hated every minute of training, but I said, 'don't quit, suffer now and live the rest of your life as a champion.'"

7. **You will have bad performances, even when you are doing all the right things.** American gymnast and Olympic gold medalist, Gabby Douglas, said, "Hard days are the best because that's where champions are made. If you push through the hard days you can get through anything."

8. **There will be days you are upset with your coach, trainer, team, and entourage.** Homer Rice, former American football player, coach, and college athletics administrator, successfully developed and implemented the Total Person Program, which is now the model for NCAA Life Skills Program currently in place in universities throughout the nation. Rice said, "You can motivate by fear, and you can motivate by reward. But both those methods are only temporary. The only lasting motivation is self-motivation."

9. **You will build many relationships and friendships that can last a lifetime.** During the 1996 Olympic Games Opening Ceremony, President of the International Olympic Committee, Juan Antonio Samaranch said, "Sport is friendship. Sport is health. Sport is education. Sport is life. Sport brings the world together."

10. **In the end, you will look back and be thankful for those who were tough and who instilled discipline in you.** You'll realize this because they really cared about you. American college basketball coach, Tom Izzo, said, "Discipline is the highest form of love. If you really love someone, you have to give them the level of discipline they need."

\* \* \*

*"Success is a journey, not a destination.*
*The doing is often more important than the outcome."*

- Arthur Ashe

# How Far Are You Willing To Go?

*The champion minded are willing to do what others aren't.*

As a kid, I wasn't the most talented or skilled athlete. When it came to captains choosing their teams, I was never the first pick. But, I learned very early in life that if I wanted to be a success, I had to work harder and to give more effort than the next guy. I also learned that it didn't just come down to who had the best skill set, but rather, to who was willing to consistently put in the extra work and to do what others weren't willing to do.

I knew that in order to make my national team and to compete in the world championships, I had to surpass my competitors' training methods. Call me obsessed, but my days started with a 4 am wake up to get in a 2 hour bike ride before work. My lunchtimes consisted of an hour gym session. After work, I'd run for 1-2 hours. This was my choice. I was willing to give the effort and to make the commitment. Some view these choices as sacrifices, but I don't see it that way. I've heard athletes talk about the sacrifices they made to get to where they are now, but when you make a choice, you are choosing to do what it takes to get you where you want to go. It's your choice. No one is - or should be - forcing you to do it.

Kobe Bryant, the NBA All-star player said it best,

> *At the end of the day, it doesn't come down to who has the most talent or intelligence. It*

*comes down to who is willing to make the choices that others are not willing to make. Like who is willing to shoot baskets in the dark when everyone else is sleeping? Who is willing to prepare more for an interview? Who is willing to practice their speech ten times more than anyone else? All are choices we make.*

I love what Kobe says, because it's so true. When skill and ability meet hard work and a champion mindset, that's where greatness happens. The champion minded are willing to do what others aren't wiling to do.

\* \* \*

*When you choose to challenge and push yourself to do what others aren't willing to do, then you'll have opportunities for greatness that others won't have.*

*"There's no way around the hard work. Embrace it. You have to put in the hours because there is always something you can improve. You have to put in a lot of sacrifice and effort for sometimes little reward, but you have to know that if you put in the right effort, the reward will come."*

- Roger Federer

# Character is Everything

*"Be more concerned with your character than your reputation, because your character is what your really are, while your reputation is merely what others think you are." –John Wooden*

Recently, I was speaking with a highly respected college coach in Florida about his recruiting process. The word character kept coming up. His strategy was simple. First, he invited the player's mother to attend the first interview with the player. He then observed the interaction between the player and his mother. No matter how talented or brilliant the player might be, if the player displayed disrespect toward their mother, the interview was over. There are many talented players, but good character is hard to find. You can teach game skills, but to teach character can be a challenge, especially as individuals age and behaviors and attitudes are deeply ingrained.

Character development and player development go hand-in-hand. The mighty All Blacks Rugby team subscribes to this when they say, "good people make good All Blacks."

## 6 pillars of good character:

1. **Trustworthiness** - Be honest. Be reliable. Do what you say you are going to do. Have the courage to do the right thing. Be loyal.

2. **Respect** - Follow the Golden Rule. Be tolerant and accepting of differences. Use good manners and good language. Be polite and considerate.

3. **Responsibility** - Plan ahead. Be diligent. Persevere. Do your best. Be self-disciplined. Be accountable for your words, actions, and attitudes. Set an example for others.

4. **Fairness** - Play by the rules. Take turns and share. Be open-minded. Listen. Don't blame others. Treat all people fairly and equally.

5. **Caring** - Be kind. Be compassionate and show empathy. Express gratitude. Help others.

6. **Citizenship** - Give back to your community. Mentor younger players. Volunteer.

\* \* \*

*"I believe ability can get you to the top, but it takes character to keep you there."*

- John Wooden

# Success is a Choice

*Champion minded athletes make choices that lead to success.*

There's just no way around it - success takes consistency and hard work. By making good choices, you take positive steps in the right direction everyday to earn you a slight edge. Your commitment to making good choices impacts how far you will go. Aim to get a little bit better - just 1% better - everyday, and you're on your way to making your vision and goals come true. Listed below are some questions to the choices you'll come across:

- Do you perform your warm up routine without coach telling you to?

- Do you make excuses or blame the weather, condition of the facility, coach, equipment, opponent, referee, teammates, spectators, officials, format of play, etc. for your losses?

- Do you surround yourself with people who inspire you and challenge you to be better?

- Do you arrive early for practice?

- Do you get enough sleep?

- Do you pack your bag and prepare your equipment the night before, or do you scramble around at the last minute?

- Do you put in extra work on your own time?

- Do you keep a journal and record your daily activities?

- Do you have a deep desire to improve and to ask questions?

- Do you help with practice by assisting the coach and other teammates?

- Do you make healthy food and drink choices?

- Do you cut corners or cheat on repetitions when coach isn't looking?

- Do you practice positive self-talk?

- Do you display positive body language?

\* \* \*

*"Parties won't take me to where I want to go."*

- Kevin Johnson, NBA Basketball player

*You are not born a winner.*
*You are not born a loser.*
*You are born a chooser.*

# Be Coachable

*The best players are open to listening and learning.*

Being coachable is not just a willingness to learn. It's a willingness to unlearn and to re-learn, which involves change. Coach-ability is a capacity that allows an individual to accept criticism, to acknowledge error, and to adapt to new information. Essential in personal and professional relationships, coach-ability is highly relevant beyond the athletic field. College coaches recruit coachable athletes. Businesses recruit coachable employees.

*An un-coachable athlete is an individual who feels that he/she is never wrong and whenever given any kind of critical or constructive feedback refuses to take responsibility for his/her mistakes or failure.* The un-coachable athlete makes excuses and redirects blame to anyone and anything but themselves. They are incurious and impenetrable. They bristle at criticism. They are consumed with self-importance or self-doubt. They refuse the gift of guidance.

When Steve Kerr, coach of the San Francisco Warriors, was asked what his star player, NBA MVP Stephen Curry's greatest asset was, he replied "coach-ability." Coach-ability is the readiness to be corrected and to act on correction. Coachable players are accountable players. They step-up and take ownership of and responsibility for their decisions and actions. To be coachable, prepare to be wrong. More opportunities come to those who are willing to listen and be taught.

## Traits of a Coachable Athlete:

1. *Humility.* No matter how much you achieve, humility allows you to stay teachable.

2. *Awareness of Purpose.* Being aware of the greater purpose of feedback creates space for improvement. Being respectful of and grateful for those giving feedback, who care about you and who want the best for you, are ways to display awareness.

3. *Trust.* Athletes who refuse to give up control until they see results, don't get the results they seek because they do not trust the process. Results come when athlete surrenders control and trusts the process.

* * *

*Coachable athletes crave feedback. They want to be told what can be better.*

*A coachable athlete is humble, disciplined and open to criticism and feedback. No matter how great they become, they still remain committed to their own personal development.*

# Discipline & Self-Control

*Champion minded athletes embrace discipline.*

To excel in anything, you need to have a high level of discipline. High achievement does not happen without discipline. The discipline to commit to what needs to be done everyday, consistently, and with great effort, is a separating factor between the good and the great athletes. Discipline is not a punishment, but rather, it urges you on when you would rather stay in the comfort of your bed. Discipline propels you on when you would rather go home, but instead, you stay and put in a little extra practice after the session ends. Discipline compels you to choose what's hard over what's easy.

By personal choice, the champion minded athlete is disciplined. Champions understand that instant gratification and laziness are the enemies of long-term success. Discipline involves more than the physical demands - it is essential to mental and emotional toughness. It takes discipline to control emotions, to follow the routines put in place to stay calm and focused and to maintain a positive attitude and confident body language. Losing control of your temper, displaying negative body language and frustration all waste your own energy and give your opponent a boost of confidence and energy. The champion minded athlete is disciplined in performing routines to stay focused on the present moment, to let go of what has already happened, and to not worry about the future. Champion minded athletes are disciplined in their routines to keep emotions under control, conserve energy, and project confidence.

The champion minded athlete takes ownership of his or her game - schedule, preparation, training, practicing, competing, nutrition/hydration, and recovery. Discipline includes doing the things you don't like to do, with a great attitude. Discipline yourself so others don't have to.

* * *

*"The definition of discipline is to do what you're supposed to do when you're supposed to do it."*

- Jim Larranaga

# Find the Right Coach

*The right coach builds people, not only skills.*

Finding the right coach is incredibly important. A great coach should teach game skills and life skills. Choosing a coach based on the successes of other athletes in the program is a common mistake. Be careful to choose the right coach for you!

Have a look at their culture, values, and principles. Find out the philosophies emphasized in the program. Do they include personal development, skilled instruction, and decision-making? Does the program nurture a love of the game? Do they have high standards? Does the coach use a command-style approach or guided-discovery? Does the coach have a culture that promotes a healthy learning environment? Most importantly, does the coach educate beyond the game, teaching life skills in addition to sport skills?

Athletes: when choosing a coach, remember you aren't only buying into their knowledge of the game, but into their mindset and their beliefs too. Choose carefully! Communication between you and your coach is vital. You have to be able to be honest with each other, to ask questions, and to be comfortable discussing everything from goals, to health, to training schedules and more.

Don't choose the best coach. Choose the RIGHT coach. One that cares about you.

\* \* \*

M

*Remember, when choosing a coach, you aren't only buying into their knowledge of the game, but their mindset and beliefs too.*

*Choose carefully!*

# You Become a Product of Your Environment

*Great cultures and work environments come down to the right people.*

The environment in which you choose to work and train is one of the most important decisions you will make in your athletic career. The great W. Clement Stone said, "You are a product of your environment." So choose the environment that will best develop you toward your objective. Analyze your life in terms of its environment. Are the things around you helping you toward success, or are they holding you back?"

It's important to remember that the people and environment you choose to have around you, affects how good or bad your habits become. You will always notice that the athletes who are dedicated to the process are thriving in an environment that is committed to the process. Training in a space in which discipline and standards are high, and where you are surrounded by like-minded people, is of tremendous benefit. Champion minded people surround themselves with other champion minded people.

Considering training environments, how modern, new, or fancy the facility is matters little. Surrounding yourself with the right people, who will help and support you along your journey, matters a lot. Through the years, I've visited some of the most simple, modest, and unremarkable training facilities in Eastern Europe and Africa. They have produced world-class athletes through high-quality coaching techniques and favorable training environments.

The main difference between these and luxury facilities was in their superior work ethic and culture. Favorable training environments have to have the right people. In Baltimore, under the leadership of influential coach Bob Bowman, one facility produced multiple Olympians and record breakers. Bowman is the long-time coach of Olympic gold-medalist Michael Phelps. Considering the number of champions that have come out of his program, it's easy to understand the importance of total immersion in a winning culture and environment. These athletes are around other champions who encourage and push each other every day.

\* \* \*

*You will always notice that the athletes who are dedicated to the process are thriving in an environment that is committed to the process.*

*The training environments you choose and the people you surround yourself with, are probably the two most important decisions you can make as an athlete.*

# Poor Quality Eventually Costs More

*Choosing the cheap choice first leads to paying more in the end.*

To be an elite athlete, one requires a good support team. Frequently, I've had a new student who has had poor quality instruction come to train with me and we initially have to spend time breaking bad habits, rebuilding fundamentals, and establishing good habits. Even though the initial instruction may have been cheaper, it lacked quality, and so the time we spent undoing what was previously done ended up costing more than the initial expense. I understand that most people do not operate on a millionaire's budget, but if you are going to pursue instruction, make sure it is fundamentally sound. Legendary Coach John Wooden famously said, "If you don't have time to do it right, when will you have time to do it over?"

Champion minded athletes seek the best coaches and the best trainers to guide their technical, tactical, physical, mental, and emotional development. It comes with a price. Usually, when you choose the cheap option, you get a lesser quality product. If you truly want to have the best, you may have to travel a longer distance and pay a higher rate; but, in the long run in will be worth it!

As Warren Buffett so famously said, "the best investment you can make is in yourself." So, don't go cheap on yourself.

\* \* \*

*Choosing the cheapest, most convenient help eventually leads to paying more, as you'll end up having to do it all over again.*

# Goal-Setting

*Set goals like an Olympian.*

Goal-setting is important. When I sit down with an athlete to discuss goals, I like to look four years ahead; as the Olympic Games happen once every four years. For an Olympic athlete to plan to train, to perform, to stay healthy, and then to peak during the Games takes serious attention to the process of setting, monitoring, and accomplishing the stated goals. This process helps you assess your current skill level, and the steps needed to progress toward the long-term goal.

## Types of Goals:

**Long-Term goals** relate to the big picture, ranging from making the high school team or travel squad, earning a college scholarship, earning a starting position, winning a conference championship, making the transition from amateur to professional, winning a major title, becoming an Olympian, to winning an Olympic gold medal for your country. These types of outcome goals serve as motivation to help you stay on track, but you actually have very little control over the external factors that affect these types of goals.

**Performance goals** are broken into specific categories mainly dealing with competition, such as developing primary and secondary patterns of play and being able to effectively apply them, improving mental and emotional control, and developing and implementing routines to better handle pressure situations.

**Process goals** encompass the daily tasks that connect the performance goals to the outcome goals. These include improving specific areas of physical skill (speed, strength, endurance, etc.), mastering fundamental techniques, developing warm-up and cool-down routines, understanding tactical plans and being able to assess and to make necessary adjustments.

Dr. Steven Ungerleider, founding board member of the Foundation for Global Sports Development and sports psychologist, says, "Since Olympians are very focused and disciplined, it was usually easy to write out a visualization plan, how to do it, when, practice, and implementation. Usually, athletes reported good short-term and long-term results."

\* \* \*

*Champion minded athletes are goal-oriented. They set long-term goals, performance goals, and process goals.*

# S.M.A.R.T. Goals

*Goals should be specific, measurable, attainable, relevant, and time specific.*

1. **Write it down.** Write your goals in the present tense and use affirmative language. Instead of saying, "I won't sleep in," say, "I will wake up at 6:00 a.m. every morning."

2. **Measure it.** Keep track of your success. This is one area where keeping a journal is very beneficial. If your goal is to arrive earlier for practice, keep track of what time you need to leave for practice to arrive at the desired time.

3. **Set deadlines.** Give yourself time limits to reach certain goals. Keep track of your progress and celebrate small victories. It might be getting your mile time down to a certain speed, or mastering a fundamental technique. Set a deadline and do what it takes to meet the deadline.

4. **Identify complications**. Complications could be a school trip, a family vacation, an injury, illness, a change in location, a change in financial budget, etc. It would be great if we could nicely and neatly go about the business of achieving our goals, but, there will always be unforeseen circumstances to interrupt progress.

5. **Overcome complications.** A few years ago I was working with an athlete and we were making great progress. Then, just before a big tournament, I changed jobs and moved to a different home. For me as the coach, and for her as my student, it was an incredibly difficult time. We found ways around the complication

by traveling to meet each other and to train on weekends. We frequently used FaceTime technology to talk to each other. Her parents would record video on a phone or a tablet and send to me for review. We made it work. Although I am no longer her primary coach, we are still in touch. I love that technology allows me to continue to be involved and to be a part of her journey.

* * *

*The champion minded set goals for the long-term, but are focused on the daily process of achieving excellence.*

# Imbalances

*Where they are priorities,*
*there will be imbalances.*

How can you maintain a balanced life while pursuing excellence? It's simple - you can't. Being aware of the areas which receive less attention when the focus shifts heavily to one particular area, can help you find greater balance. Doing so helps you maintain a measure of perspective. Perfect balance is unlikely, but, measuring the following 7 essentials, will help you stay on track and avoid burn out. When you measure, a score of 1 is the least amount of energy devoted and a score of 10 is the most amount of energy devoted.

1. **Family**. Are you spending time with family - parents, siblings, spouse, kids, extended family - how would you measure your family time? Family relationships are essential. You need your family for support, and they need you too. When you are an elite athlete, there will be times when you miss family functions, but do try to prioritize family.

2. **Spiritual**. This means different things to different people, including: reading inspirational passages to start your day, spending time in nature, or attending church. Do you spend time in prayer? Do you meditate? We need to connect with something greater than ourselves. We need renewal. We need rest. We need spiritual connection. Find a way to make time, even if only a few minutes, for your spirit.

3. **Community**. How are you giving back? What are you doing to contribute to your community? How do you show gratitude? There is great reward in giving to and serving others. Between practice, training, traveling, and competition, the elite athlete's schedule doesn't leave much time for volunteering. Still, there are ways to give back within your sport. Make time to help a younger player, or help coaches by setting up and breaking down the practice gear. Even small acts like picking up trash to help keep a facility clean is an act of service.

4. **Health**. As an athlete, this one should be very high up on the scale. It's on the list because we all need to take care of our health. We need to be mindful of what we eat and drink and of how much we exercise. When striving to reach the elite levels of sport, this area is always out of balance, tipping to the high side of the scale. Reaching the highest levels of sport requires more attention to health than for your average person.

5. **Financial**. What does your budget look like? Chances are, if you're an elite athlete, this is also out of balance. Training, coaching, traveling, equipment - the life of an elite athlete comes with a price tag. It's important to be aware of financial costs, but be careful not to let your finances add pressure to your performance. I once overheard a parent tell her 12 year old daughter, "You better do well this weekend. It's costing us a fortune to be here!" We should all try to live within our means; however, it's more challenging when you're trying to reach the elite levels of sport.

6. **Social**. We all need social interaction. To be successful, you need a strong support team. Beyond family and coaches, this extends to your friends. My mom always told me that in order to have good friends, I needed to be a good friend - to be there

for them, to listen, and to support them if I wanted them to be there to listen and to support me. This can be a challenge for elite athletes. The training and competing schedule is demanding. The nutrition and hydration requirements are limiting. There will be times you miss out on social events, but this doesn't mean you can't be social.

7. **Business**. If you're a student-athlete, you have two businesses: academics and athletics. There's no way around it. To be competitive at the highest levels of sport you have to put an incredible amount of time and energy to get there and to stay there. However, education is also highly important. You also need to prepare for life after your athletic career.

Reviewing this list of basic necessities, it becomes very clear that elite athlete or not, there is no way to attend to each of these areas to create a perfectly balanced life. *It's not possible.* It is possible to keep a check on your list and to do your best to balance out the scale.

\* \* \*

*When you are aiming for excellence,*
*there will be imbalances.*

# Can't

*Eliminate the word can't from your vocabulary.*

My athletes are forbidden to use the word *can't*. The word *can't* limits, weakens, and depletes you. It sabotages the strength and resilience you need to conquer the obstacles and challenges in front of you.

What we say to ourselves on a daily basis can have an enormous affect on our lives. The words you think will shape your life. Our words mold us and we eventually become them. *Can't* doesn't resonate with a champion minded mentality.

The most decorated swimmer and Olympian of all time, Michael Phelps, said that when he first started to train with his coach, he was forbidden to say the word *can't,* so that he could broaden his mind and believe he could achieve whatever he wanted to.

Mike Norton, a 7-time winner of the USS Dwight Eisenhower award said it best,

> *Never say that you can't do something, or that something seems impossible, or that something can't be done, no matter how discouraging or harrowing it may be; human beings are limited only by what we allow ourselves to be limited by: our own minds. We are each the masters of our own reality; when we become self-aware to this: absolutely anything in the world is possible.*

M

Starting today, eliminate the word *can't* from your vocabulary. Empower yourself with words that make you feel unstoppable.

\* \* \*

*Turn your "can't do's" into "can do's" and watch how things dramatically start to change for the better.*

# Believe You Can!

*Failure brings you closer to success.*

Today is a gift. Make the best of today by not looking back. Looking back only serves to hold you back. When you are focused on today and giving your very best, you set yourself up to having a greater impact on tomorrow.

Swedish and Manchester United soccer star, Zlatan Ibrahimovic grew up in the ghetto of Malmö, Sweden. With a Bosnian father and Croatian mother, his family was discriminated against because of their immigrant status. At age 15, he considered quitting his football career to work the docks in Malmö. His manager convinced him to continue playing, and having won 32 trophies in his career, he has gone on to be the second most decorated active footballer in the world as of February 2017.

Knowing that every failure experienced along the way ultimately brings them closer to success, champion minded athletes persist. You are not defined by where you are from, who your parents/ancestors are, or what was done in the past. You choose your goals. You choose your attitude and actions. You choose your future! When he was growing up, Ibrahimovic idolized Brazilian star Ronaldo. He had a dream and a vision, and he was fortunate to have a manager to encourage him to pursue his dream. After being on the brink of giving up, he persisted on and never looked back! Zlatan had the attitude and mindset of "If it's meant to be, it's up to me."

Champion minded athletes have a vision, commit to a goal, surround themselves with the right people, and persist through failure. Never let someone tell you you can't!

* * *

*Belief is a state of mind. Beliefs drive behavior, and behaviors affect performance.*

*Never let any person, any obstacle, any doubt, any fear or negative voice, keep you from becoming who you want to be.*

# True Self-Confide

*Champion minded athletes trust their abilities, qualities, and judgement.*

As an athlete, true self-confidence doesn't merely help you perform better on the court, field, or track, it also allows you to see and to accept yourself exactly as you are. Sometimes what we perceive as confidence is actually a sign of arrogance. Two-time British Olympian track runner and a good friend of mine, Jack Green, put it beautifully when he said, "True self confidence isn't loud, it's silent."

True self-confidence is about being comfortable in your skin, recognizing your strengths as well as your weaknesses. It allows you to appreciate the skills and the talents you have, as well as the qualities that have gotten you to where you are today. Jack added, "True self-confidence is having a humility and appreciation for the work you've put in."

When you are truly self-confident, you know you cannot be great at everything. With true self-confidence, you recognize your shortcomings, your weaknesses, and your past failures without the need to hide or to beat yourself up. If you have true self-confidence, you are committed to continual improvement in the areas in which you may already excel, while also developing those areas in which you are not as strong.

In life you will face many setbacks. One of the many advantages of building true self-confidence is the ability to persevere through the inevitable up and downs you will face. These will occur in your sports career and in your life. To become truly self-confident, you first need to personally reflect, to take a good hard look at yourself. Through self-reflection, you will accept that setbacks are a part of life, and that some disappointment is inevitable. By embracing the principles of self-reflection and the ability to look deep within (not always easy), you'll find the place where the greatest change happens.

With true self-confidence, you are able to gain a healthy and balanced perspective. Too often in the sports world, I consult with athletes who carry the burden of feeling they are being judged by their results. How well we kick, throw, or hit a ball does not determine our self-worth. Self-worth derives from how we embrace the journey of life, the difficulties within, and how we overcome them.

In the end, true self-confidence comes down to self-acceptance: the good, the bad, and the ugly. It's a mindset of getting up in the morning and aiming to become not just a better athlete, but a better person. It's about seeing self-improvement as a life long journey. And that is something to be fully excited about and invested in for life!

# Overcoming Adversity

*Any great athlete who has reached the top
has overcome adversity.*

A few years ago I attended a basketball coaches' conference in Las Vegas, Nevada which included a stay at the Hard Rock Café Hotel & Casino as part of the package for coaches. While there, I observed all the memorabilia of past and present musicians and artists ranging from the Beatles, to Jimmy Hendrix, to Britney Spears. One piece in particular intrigued me - the drum set from the rock band, Def Leppard.

It is one of the most fascinating contraptions I have ever seen! The drum set was modified to accommodate the drummer, Rick Allen, who had lost an arm in a near-fatal car accident. The drum set was designed for him to play with his feet and one arm. In an interview for *Modern Drummer*, Allen had this to say, "not being able to play again never really crossed my mind... it's like anything, when you're thrown in at the deep end, you really have to swim, and this was a classic case of having to do that. I don't think I ever doubted that I could do it. I was just being as positive as I could." Interested in learning more, I researched Allen and how he came back from the devastating accident to re-teach himself how to play the drums and to continue performing at a high level.

After consulting various drum-set builders to design a set that would accommodate his needs, he was determined to play again. When asked if he's always been so determined, he replied, "Going through what I did made me a stronger person, but if you knew the rest of the guys, you would understand why. Def Leppard is a very close-knit unit — not just the band, but everybody concerned with it. Everybody was just saying, 'Come on now, Rick. You can do it.'" With determination, drive, self-belief, and support from those around him, Allen adapted and learned to perform at an even higher level than he had played previously. Def Leppard became a multi-platinum album selling band with earnings over $200 million.

When it comes to sports, adversity can come in many forms - through injury, defeat, or being dropped from the team. How we handle and overcome these challenges determines our rate of success. In Rick Allen's case, his positive attitude proved to be the foundation of his ability to overcome adversity.

* * *

*It's our attitude when dealing with adversity that determines our level of success.*

# Are You Accountable?

*"Responsibility equals accountability equals ownership." –Pat Summitt*

Defining characteristics of champion minded athletes include: responsibility, accountability, and ownership. Being responsible means exercising self-control and discipline. Being accountable is how you justify your decisions and your actions. Taking ownership means leading, managing, and being in command of your decisions and actions.

Many former athletes will tell you that a sports career can be very short. Most will play as children and throughout their youth. Some will continue during their college years and very few will go on to compete professionally. Even the best professionals rarely have careers beyond 35 years of age (besides sports such as Golf, Motorsports, etc). With this in mind, it's important to develop the life skills of responsibility, accountability, and ownership. Former tennis great Andre Agassi once said, "We spend one third of our lives not really preparing for the other two thirds. After a sports career, there's a whole new other life to manage."

Before I begin working with an athlete, I make my standards and my expectations clear. By giving them a significant role in the management of their own daily activities and tasks, I involve the athlete 100%. Not only is the individual accountable to themselves, they also understand their decisions and actions affect the people around them – coaches, teammates, parents, etc. If the athlete falls short of the standards, and/or fails to meet expectations, they are not only hurting themselves, but they are also letting others down. These are important life lessons.

When college coaches assess new recruits, they look for individuals who are accountable. Former NBA coach Lenny Wilkens once said, "The most important quality I look for in a player is accountability. You've got to be accountable for who you are. It's too easy to blame things on someone else."

Responsibility, accountability, and ownership expose themselves when the athlete is on their own with no coach, parent, nor teammate present. Champion minded athletes take it upon themselves to be prepared for competition. They know what needs to be done, and they make sure they do what is necessary to be ready. Former legendary women's basketball coach Pat Summitt said it best, "Responsibility equals accountability equals ownership. And a sense of ownership is the most powerful weapon a team or an individual can have."

\* \* \*

*"The most important quality I look for in a player is accountability."*

– Lenny Wilkens

*Discipline yourself so someone else doesn't have to – it's a form of accountability. The more accountable you become, the more disciplined in life you will become.*

*When you are tough on yourself, life becomes easier on you.*

# Attitude & Self-Talk

*Your attitude and self-talk are your choice.*

Champions consistently choose the right attitude. They understand and believe that to be an elite performer they must consciously choose positivity. All else being equal between two opponents, the one who triumphs is the one who chooses a winning attitude and mindset.

There is no substitute for being coachable. Being coachable is directly linked to attitude and mindset. Both are choices reflected by behavior. How coachable you are has a significant effect on your performances and results. If you want to be great, you need to be willing and able to hear and to follow instructions. A champion minded athlete commits to listening and to observing with a humble and open mind. Choosing a positive attitude and mindset changes your perspective on the grind, and changes how you respond to challenges.

I'm privileged to work with some of the best athletes in the world, but I feel equally privileged to work with many aspiring young athletes as well. I strongly believe that a young athlete's progress depends much more on a good attitude than on physical skill. Training attitude, mindset, and coach-ability in the early ages and stages of an athlete's development are fundamental to learning and growth.

The attitude you choose everyday, and the quality of your self-talk are two of the most powerful methods to gaining confidence. Psychologist Susan Krauss Whitbourne, Ph.D. describes self-talk:

"When it is upbeat and self-validating, the results can boost your productivity. However, when the voice is critical and harsh, the effect can be emotionally crippling."

Attitude, mindset, self-talk, and a willingness to learn are personal choices. Choose your standards, abide by them daily, trust them, and then watch your confidence dramatically increase. When you dedicate yourself to higher standards and to a winning attitude on a daily basis, you begin to see positive results happen in your life.

\* \* \*

*"A bad attitude is worse than a bad swing."*

\- Payne Stewart, former U.S. Open Golf Champion

# Gratification: Now vs Later

*Stay patient yet persistent in the pursuit of excellence.*

Champion minded athletes understand the importance of putting off instant gratification and staying disciplined in pursuit of the bigger, future prize. These athletes know that the difference between looking at the small picture versus the big picture is to embrace the journey; the triumphs and the defeats along the way. Former world number one golfer, Jason Day, sums it up saying, "So many players get impatient and don't embrace the everyday process. They want results quickly. To be at the top level in this sport, or any other sport for that matter, you need to be able to endure the boring stuff and do that consistently well everyday."

Instant gratification is the enemy of hard work and patience. Focusing on the bigger picture, and looking long term, requires a willingness to fail along the way. Many athletes want to win now and miss out on the opportunity to get better and to develop. Champion minded athletes know that they will have to make changes - some big, some small - along the way to success. Usually, when a change is made, performance gets worse before it gets better. Athletes focused on immediate results are unwilling to miss shots and to lose games due to a change that will prove beneficial later. Champion minded athletes are willing to lose in the short term in order to stay on track for long term success.

In their pursuit of excellence, champion minded athletes are patient and persistent. They commit to daily habits that work toward the greater goal. Champion minded athletes resist the temptation to demand immediate results. They work hard to achieve great long-term results. They have a vision of the future and they are willing to stay focused and dedicated to the process.

* * *

*The champion minded athlete embraces the everyday process.*

# 10 Traits of Growth & Fixed Mindsets

*Champion minded athletes
display the traits of a growth mindset.*

## Growth Mindset Athletes:

1. Embrace challenges, look to improve, and to develop new skills

2. Learn from feedback and criticism, appreciate and welcome guidance, are coachable

3. Believe intelligence and talent can be developed through dedication and hard work

4. Give more effort, enjoy the battle

5. Keep trying and never give up, even when success takes time

6. Persist in the face of adversity and maintain a positive attitude

7. Are inspired by the success of others, cheer for others, are willing to help others

8. View failure as an opportunity to learn and to improve, are accountable and responsible

9. Commit to long-term development and hard work over time to achieve goals

10. Continue to learn, value innovative ideas

## Fixed Mindset Athletes:

1. Avoid challenges, prefer to do what they are already good at doing

2. Do not listen to feedback or accept criticism, become defensive, are not coachable

3. Believe intelligence and talent are set and unchanging

4. Give less effort, expect and prefer easy victories

5. Give up easily, especially when success is not immediate

6. Surrender in the face of adversity, have a defeatist attitude

7. Are threatened by the success of others, hope for others to fail, are unwilling to give back

8. View failure as a defining characteristic, make excuses and place blame

9. Are not willing to commit to long-term development, seek immediate and easy success

10. Are not interested in new, progressive ideas, see no value in continuing education

# Ways to Develop a Growth Mindset

## *Champion minded athletes are comfortable being uncomfortable.*

**Give your best effort** - Champion minded athletes focus on the process and effort that lead to success. Be aware of how hard you are trying. Praise your own good efforts. Keep trying.

**Adapt** - Champion minded athletes are aware of which strategies are working and which are not working, and they are willing and able to make necessary changes. Rather than continually making the same mistakes, they ask themselves, "what can I do differently?" and they are willing to try different strategies.

**Focus on performance rather than results** - Champion minded athletes view competition as a test of skill and knowledge, both of which can be developed and improved. Fixed mindset athletes view competition as a comparison of ultimate ability. Whereas fixed mindset athletes focus on results (ego-oriented), champion minded athletes focus on performance (task-oriented). Champion minded athletes are task-oriented. They are intrinsically motivated, confident, disciplined, and determined. Athletes - focus your mindset on learning, improving, and developing rather than on outscoring an opponent.

**Persist** - In spite of difficulty or opposition, champion minded athletes keep trying. Persistence is a key life skill. Champion minded athletes don't quit when circumstances become challenging. When faced with adversity, champion minded athletes persist.

**Get comfortable being uncomfortable** - Champion minded athletes push themselves past their limits in order to extend their limits. Champion minded athletes are willing to get out of their comfort zone and to make mistakes. This takes courage and curiosity. Athletes with a fixed mindset believe making mistakes signals incompetence. They are afraid of looking bad, and so they choose to play it safe, staying within their comfort zones. Learning is messy. Skills often get worse before they get better. Athletes - be willing to make mistakes. Fear of looking bad stunts growth and leads to lesser performance. Playing it safe doesn't lead to improvement. Challenge yourself.

**Be inspired** - On May 6, 1954, Roger Bannister became the first human to run a sub-four minute mile. At the time, it was considered an impossible feat. Runners had come close for decades, but no one had passed the mark. Bannister's accomplishment opened the door for runner after runner to also beat the four-minute mark. The power of Bannister's belief enabled him to accomplish more than what was previously thought possible. Inspired by his success, others went on to achieve their own. The success of others inspires champion minded athletes and they use it as motivation to better themselves.

# Energy Takers vs Energy Givers

## *Protect your energy.*

There are two kinds of people in this world - energy takers and energy givers. When you enter a room for a formal business meeting, a party, a presentation, a casual gathering of friends, there is an energy in the space. It can be positive or negative, warm or cold, welcoming or uninviting, tense or relaxed, festive or restrained, celebratory or dejected, etc. The same applies to meeting someone for the first time. People have an aura, which affects the greeting.

Energy directly relates to success. I'm very protective of my own energy. It's sacred to me. Your happiness and well-being are part of your energy. Recognizing its importance, champion minded athletes nurture and protect their energy.

Energy givers are those people who you are easily attracted to. Being around them, you feel enlivened and rejuvenated. They brighten any room and just the sight of them can be inspiring. They are more interested in others than themselves. They ask questions and they listen more than they talk. They are cheerful, enthusiastic, encouraging, and thoughtful. Energy givers leave a positive impact on everyone they encounter.

Energy takers are negative and self-centered. They are cynical, defeatist, gloomy, fatalistic, critical, disinterested and dismissive. Energy takers are like leeches. Spending time with energy takers leaves you exhausted and disheartened. They have a problem for every solution. Avoid them at all costs. Although you may want to do so, it's not your duty to "convert" the energy takers, because most of the time they actually want to stay in that place!

Champion minded athletes are energy givers and they surround themselves with energy givers too. They nurture and protect their own energy.

\* \* \*

*There are two types of people in this world –*
*the energy takers and the energy givers.*
*Surround yourself with those who energize you,*
*not those who suck the life out of you.*

# Entitlement is a Disease

*Be grateful.*
*Don't expect special privileges or favors.*

ntitlement is currently an epidemic, and it has infected athletes from the professional arena to the junior ranks. Entitlement is defined as the belief that one is inherently deserving of privileges or special treatment. All too often, a young athlete will excel in a particular sport and then receive special treatment. One of the biggest contributing factors to a child feeling entitled is adults, especially parents, who place the child on a pedestal. By giving special treatment to those who are successful at a sport, society has fueled entitlement among young athletes. When it comes to competitive sports, this is where I believe society is broken. Athletes then perceive themselves as outside or above the rules, deserving of special favor.

By instilling a fixed mindset, feelings of entitlement limit an athlete's progress. These athletes make an art form of excuse-making. They look to place blame. They give up easily. David Carter, of the USC Sports Business Institute explains that a large part of the current culture of entitlement has been cultivated from very early ages, "We all know of the stage parents and the culture of youth sports, which is affecting and infecting these kids at a much younger age than it used to. Now it's all about club sports and making the traveling team and parents wanting to get their children into position to secure a college scholarship earlier." Anyone who has been to a youth sporting event is familiar with the showboating or petulant child and the accommodating, adoring parents.

## Entitlement can manifest itself in a variety of ways:

- A lack of consequences for inappropriate behavior.
- A feeling of deserving special treatment.
- A belief that the rules do not apply to the athletes.
- A disregard for authority coupled with feelings of superiority.

Recognizing and rewarding athletic success, without also acknowledging the importance of character, sets a dangerous precedent. Athletes: you are more than your athletic prowess. You are not defined by what you do, but rather by who you are are. If you have been given the gift of natural talent, what are you doing to give back? Be grateful and remember to regularly thank your parents, coaches, trainers, and supporters for helping you reach your goals.

* * *

*Gratitude is an attitude, and so is entitlement.*
*Both are a choice.*

# Champion Minded vs Average Minded

*Whether you think you can,*
*or you think you can't; you're right.*

## Champion Minded Athletes:

1. Believe they have what it takes to succeed

2. Have a tireless work ethic

3. Have a positive attitude and uplifting energy

4. Choose to do the extra work

5. Are intrinsically motivated

6. Are humble and honest

7. Have affirmative, encouraging self-talk

8. Do what's right even when no one is watching

9. Never give up

10. Are accountable

## Average Minded Athletes:

1. Lack self-belief and are encumbered by self-doubt

2. Give effort based on how they feel that day

3. Have a negative attitude and burdensome energy

4. Only do the bare minimum of what is asked

5. Take no ownership or initiative

6. Feel entitled

7. Have critical, fatalistic self-talk

8. Slack off when coach is away

9. Quit when challenged

10. Make excuses, place blame, and complain

*"Champions behave like champions before they're champions; they have a winning standard of performance before they are winners."*

- Bill Walsh

# SECTION 2:

# *Learning to Train*

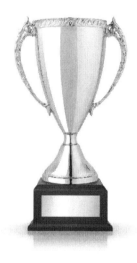

# Desire

*"Desire is the starting point of all achievement."*
*–Napoleon Hill*

## Champion minded athletes desire:

1. to get better everyday.

2. to improve their self-talk everyday.

3. to do the extra work away from set practice time.

4. to understand and to ask more.

5. to prepare better.

6. to improve their nutritional habits.

7. to improve their weaknesses and better their strengths.

8. to get to practice before time, not on time.

9. to surround themselves with the right people.

10. to master the fundamentals of the game.

11. to improve their daily lifestyle habits.

12. to spend more time in the gym getting stronger.

13. to improve their sleeping and recovery habits.

14. to embrace struggle and to meet challenges head-on.

15. to outwork their opponents every day of the week.

16. to do the small things incredibly well.

17. to bring the right attitude to practice everyday.

18. to bring their best effort to practice everyday.

19. to communicate and listen better.

20. to give back to the game and to help others less fortunate than themselves.

# What Separates the Good from the Great

*Mindset, attitude and purpose separate the good from the great.*

The best teams and individual athletes are more invested in the everyday grind. They are more committed to the extra work. They have a greater vision, passion, and purpose for what they do - a bigger drive, a greater motivation, and a *WHY*.

The best teams and individual athletes love to compete. They are driven by the challenge of pushing themselves to their limits and beyond. They get outside of their comfort zones.

The best teams and individual athletes have a growth mindset. They aren't afraid to take risks and to fail. They view mistakes and failures as opportunities to learn, to grow and to improve.

The best teams and individual athletes are problem solvers. They embrace the struggle. Because they test themselves in their training, when they are tested in competition, they are prepared to make good decisions and stay calm under pressure.

The best teams and individual athletes have great character. They have high standards. They are respectful, reliable, honest, loyal, trustworthy, and accountable.

The best teams and individual athletes have grit, resilience, and a hunger to succeed. They are willing to go harder, longer, and further than the rest.

\* \* \*

*The road to success is filled with obstacles, challenges, and disappointments. Face them, embrace them, and overcome them.*

*Successful people do not decide their future; they decide their habits and their habits decide their future.*

# Choose Your Training Environment Wisely

*Choose to train in a culture of excellence.*

T he environment in which you choose to train is of the utmost importance to your success. In fact, it's probably one of the most important decisions you can make as an athlete.

Over the years, I've discovered that so much focus is placed on the behavior change of the individual. Yet, that's only half the story. Working to build a better self almost always means working to build a better community or team around you. A big part of success involves the people with whom you choose to surround yourself.

I've always been a believer that too much luxury creates a soft mindset. Luxury creates complacency and sometimes even entitlement. Fancy training facilities, with cutting-edge technology, may be impressive, but they can also lead to an athlete feeling that they deserve special treatment or are above putting in the hard yards. Cultivating grit and developing toughness can be difficult in a cushy setting.

Great training environments begin with having the right people, a supportive community and an encouraging culture. They require a culture in which the right attitude and work ethic are present, a culture in which everyone involved demands excellence.

When you are immersed in an environment that maintains high standards and demands discipline, you absorb the energy and take that energy into performance. When the athletes and coaches are all committed to getting better everyday and supporting each other, excellence happens.

In choosing the right environment, make sure that a great energy and a positive vibe is present. You also need athletes that are as good, or even better than you, to challenge and push you. Avoid choosing an academy, club or facility based solely on past results. Choose the right one for you, one that pushes you to be better, not only as an athlete, but as a person.

When it comes to choosing your training environment, think people and culture first. To become champion minded, you need to surround yourself with champion minded people.

\* \* \*

*Choose a training environment that motivates you to work hard. One that nurtures a champion mindset.*

# Surround Yourself with the Right People

*Champion minded athletes seek out people who inspire them.*

The people with whom you surround yourself on a daily basis influence the way you think, act, and feel. Champion minded athletes surround themselves with people who inspire them and who push them to be better. They avoid people who drain their energy and who distract them from reaching their full potential.

Champion minded athletes seek out relentless workers who are passionate and committed. Athletes: it's hard to be relentless in the pursuit of excellence when the people around you slack off during practice and give up during competition. Surround yourself with people who share similar goals and work ethic.

Champion minded athletes seek people with positive attitudes. Athletes: negativity drags you down and exhausts your energy. Surround yourself with greatness; people who are optimistic, positive, and driven. Positive people help you raise your standards, inspire you, and push you on toward your vision and your goals.

Champion minded athletes seek people who are lifelong-learners. Lifelong learning is the "ongoing, voluntary, and self-motivated" quest for knowledge. Whatever your aspirations may be, find those who have reached the top and soak up their knowledge. Learn from their experience and follow their example.

The people around you matter. You need good people who will challenge you and make you better, who will raise your standards and help you maintain them. You become like the people you spend the most time with. Make sure they motivate you, inspire you, and challenge you to do and to be more. Avoid those who are content to be average. Trust that hard work, a positive attitude, and lifelong learning will help make your vision become a reality.

\* \* \*

*The people around you matter.*
*You need the right people who will challenge you*
*and make you better.*

*Trust the Process.*
*Be patient with yourself.*
*Surround yourself with good people.*
*Enjoy the journey.*

# Don't Go Cheap!

## *Champion minded athletes invest in themselves.*

In your sport and in life, there is no better investment you can make than in yourself. When you make the commitment to invest in yourself, the return on investment multiplies over time. Champion minded athletes invest in themselves. They are willing to go the extra miles to get the best support. If it means taking a long trip to visit a specialist or someone who can help their game, they do it. They are committed to finding the right people, the right team, training environment, and equipment. They are willing to do whatever it takes to get better.

Often athletes attempt go on the cheap. Understand that if you want the best, then you better be prepared to pay. As in life, if you want the best doctors, lawyers, or advisors, you are going to pay a higher price. Understandably, we don't all have the budget of a highly paid athlete, but going cheap on the contributing factors to your performance and career may end up being more costly in the end. Too often, I see athletes compromising the quality of their coaching and training in an attempt to save money. As the saying goes, "hire cheap and you will end up paying double later." Never mind the time you have wasted in the process.

Also, don't go cheap on equipment - especially the quality of shoes you wear. I've seen athletes wear a poor quality sponsor's shoe and subsequently get injured. Choosing cheaper equipment risks your health and the longevity of your career. Reaching the elite level in any sport is expensive, but cutting corners on coaching, training, and equipment can be even more costly.

The champion minded understand that to maximize your abilities and to become the best, you must be willing to acquire the best people to help you improve. It might cost you a bit now, but in the long run, the pay off and the results come back to you.

* * *

*Commit to investing in yourself. Start by finding the right people to surround yourself with.*

# Find Tough-Leaders, Not Cheerleaders

*Seek leaders who are tough, but fair.*

Champion minded athletes surround themselves with people of good character and high standards. They look for coaches and trainers who are tough but fair, who tell them what they need to hear and not just what they want to hear. Champion minded athletes are self-motivated and confident, which allows them to choose tough leaders to help them on their journey.

Champion minded athletes do not need constant affirmation or folks in their entourage to remind them of their greatness and to feed their ego. I've seen athletes, who sign a big contract or who receive a large amount of money, start to attract the "hanger-on" and "yes" people to their mix. These hangers-on and yes people are fair-weather friends, great to have around when things are going well, but who scatter when the going gets tough.

The best teachers and coaches I remember from my school days are the ones who were tough on me. Maybe I didn't fully understand it then, but now I'm so thankful and grateful for those lessons learned. It was those tough teachers and coaches who led me to places I'd never been before. They led me out of my comfort zone, demanded focus, and required total effort from me at all times.

Over years working with the most successful athletes, the commonalities shone forth. They were all highly disciplined, humble, and appreciative. These were also the ones that not only excelled in their chosen sport, but more importantly, in life too.

Champion minded athletes have a certain confidence, calmness, and self-assurance about them. Along their developmental path, tough leaders nurtured these traits.

Athletes: find tough leaders who are demanding, but fair, not cheerleaders to boost your ego. Seek people with high standards - people who have good values and principles. Find coaches who don't only seek to improve sports skills in their athletes, but who develop life skills in their athletes. Surround yourself with people who will help you stay on the right path and support you through the highs and lows.

\* \* \*

*If your coach pushes you, if your coach disciplines you, if your coach demands the best from you, then your coach truly cares about you.*

# Comfort Seekers

*Champion minded athletes seek out those who tell them what they need to hear.*

A comfort seeker is an athlete who would rather be coached by someone who tells them what they *want* to hear, rather than what they *need* to hear. Comfort seekers are athletes who do their best to avoid hard work and putting in the daily grind. They fear the truth, they seek the easy coaches, and they avoid the tough coaches who will challenge them and push them to better performance.

Comfort seekers are often talented, but lazy. They like to control their own schedules and practices, and they don't take instruction well. Put simply, they are not coachable.

Recognizing comfort seekers is easy. They make excuses and complain when a coach demands excellence. They play the victim. When it comes to poor results or form, they place blame on others, including the coach. Despite all the opportunities they've been given, they rant about life's unfairness and about how unlucky they are.

Athletes: if you do not demand the best from yourself, you are cheating yourself. Find a coach who is unafraid to speak the truth and who says what you *need* to hear. Improvement comes from learning to accept feedback and to see how it can bring you advantage. Develop grit, learn how to accept criticism and discipline yourself. Stop seeking what is *easy*. Stop taking short cuts. The world is full of *yes* people. Avoid them! They won't help you get where you want to go.

If your coach is tough, (but fair) on you - then stick with that person. Lucky you – it means they actually care about you! Believe me, one day you will thank them. These people don't come around very often in life. Endure the challenge, embrace the struggle and build some grit!

* * *

*Surround yourself with those who tell you what you NEED to hear, not only what you WANT to hear.*

# Win the Day

*Champion minded athletes focus on
taking care of today.*

A few years back, while watching the Oregon Ducks football team on television, I heard the slogan "Win the Day." In an effort to spur his players' effort during spring practices, Chip Kelly, head coach at the time, established the mantra: *Win the Day.* Each day at practice, he recognized "winners" at their respective positions. Years later, Kelly's top-ranked Oregon Ducks claimed *Win the Day* as their motto. It is splashed on a Eugene billboard, in the locker room and in giant letters on the players' entrance to Autzen Stadium. "To me, it means you take care of what you can control, and what we can control is today," Kelly said. "I think people too often look way down the road – you know, 'I want to do this, I want to do that, I want to be conference champion, national champion.' If you don't take care of Tuesday, that's not going to happen."

Champion minded athletes embrace the idea of winning the day to be able to win on the big day. Consistently having a good attitude, committing to good routines and habits, controlling the controllables, giving your best effort, putting in the extra time - these are all ways you can win the day.

Aiming to "win the day" is how you build confidence. Reach for the standards you've set each and everyday. This provides the foundation to achieve long-term goals. It's about doing your very best today and no matter how small or how great, recognizing your efforts and achievements. Acknowledge a good practice. See the improvement in a skill you've been developing. Remember a compliment given to you by a coach. Winning the day is much like building a wall. Each day you add the bricks of confidence through positive self-reflection. If you are only waiting for the wins or results to give you confidence, then you miss the vital steps needed to build it.

\* \* \*

*Building confidence is much like building a wall. Each day you are adding the bricks through positive self-reflection.*

M

# Champions Don't Sleep In

*Champion minded athletes love to get a head start on the competition.*

I've never met a successful person who regularly sleeps late. Successful people want to get their day started as early as possible. They want to get out and make things happen. Instead of lying in bed dreaming about it, they are out there doing it. Recently, I read an article in the *Wall Street Journal* that listed the most productive hours of the day to be between 4:00 a.m. and 6:00 a.m., due to a well-rested and alert mind and body, and a lack of distractions. I'm not suggesting we all need to start our day at 4:00 a.m., but rising early is an important habit that takes self-discipline. Champion minded people are early risers because they want to get a head start on their competition. It's pretty simple - those who get up early, get more done.

Champion minded athletes maximize time management. They schedule training time and recovery time into the structure of each day. When starting with a new client or athlete, one of the first steps I take is to study their daily routine. When it comes to energy management, I want to know if they're maximizing their whole day. If you are not an early riser, I encourage you to train yourself to become an early riser. Start by getting up just 15 minutes earlier and understand that you'll also need to go to bed 15 minutes earlier. Getting the proper amount of sleep is vital to performance and well-being. Structure your day to allow for 7-9 hours of sleep and rise early. It may be difficult at first, but do it until it becomes a habit.

The Champion minded are the doers, not the dreamers. They are early risers who aim to get a head start on their competition.

\* \* \*

*You can either lie in your bed and dream about it, or you can get out and make it happen!*

# Discipline Starts With Making Your Bed

*Champion minded athletes start each day with this one simple act.*

From as early as I can remember, my parents told me to make my bed first thing every morning. I didn't fully understand or appreciate it at the time, but years later I discovered the true value of this one simple act. Making the bed presents me with my first act of discipline of the day. Right from the start, I feel more productive and ready to take on the day. It's an important part of my daily routine that provides me with structure and momentum, which lead to a more confident mindset to achieve my goals for the day.

You may be thinking, "Seriously? You feel like you've accomplished something just by making your bed in the morning?" *Yes!* Anything that requires an act of discipline or service is an achievement. Athletes: how you start your day greatly impacts the rest of the day. In order to stay disciplined, create positive habits and routines.

By making my bed and keeping my room tidy, I have a clean space and a clear mind to be productive and on task. Being organized helps me to be prepared, on time, and alert. I've always believed that a messy space leads to a messy mind. I've found that a disorganized, cluttered space makes for a distracted, anxious mindset.

I also make my bed each morning because it is MY bed. Even if you enjoy the privilege of having a housekeeper or a cleaning service to keep your space neat and clean, you should still take responsibility for making your bed. I even make my bed when staying in hotels! I am forever grateful to my parents for instilling this simple act of discipline to start my day.

\* \* \*

*"If you want to change the world, start off by making your own bed."*

- Admiral William McRaven

# Lombardi Time

*Champion minded athletes value their time.*

L egendary head coach of the Green Bay Packers, Vince Lombardi, believed that in order to be on time, players needed to arrive at least 15 minutes early for practices or meetings. He held his players accountable to high standards - 10 minutes early was actually 5 minutes late. His strict time standard become known as *Lombardi Time*. Via these standards, Lombardi changed the Packers from a losing team into a Super Bowl championship team.

Manchester United's former captain, Roy Keane, was another stickler for time keeping. Under legendary coach Sir Alex Ferguson, Keane believed that the players had to be in the locker rooms 30 minutes before every practice started. In this way, players could do their usual chatting, get changed and laced up. During the late 1990's and early 2000's, Manchester United went on to become one of the most dominant forces in world football.

Champion minded athletes show up early and well-prepared. They believe in Lombardi Time. Champion minded athletes are aware that uncontrollable circumstances can arise at any time, so they plan ahead to allow for unforeseen situations. Planning ahead limits stress and anxiety, allowing for a calm and focused mindset. When rushed or running late, it takes even more time to settle down and to ready yourself. This affects performance.

Athletes: good time management skills are part of the standards you keep. Early is on time, on time is late, and late is unacceptable. Lateness reveals a lack of pride and passion for what you do. Being organized, prepared, and early communicates a high level of respect and importance. Whether it is a personal or professional appointment, being early shows that you care and are reliable. Since showing up late for a job interview or meeting can cost you dearly, being early is an important life lesson. Be champion minded in your time management and plan ahead.

\* \* \*

*Good time management skills are part of the standards you keep.*

# 86,400 Seconds in a day

## *Champion minded athletes are great time managers.*

No matter who you are, where you're from, or what you do, everyone has the same amount of time in a day: 24 hours, or 86,400 seconds. How you choose to spend your time determines your level of success.

Athletes: have you ever noticed that the people who are always saying that they're busy, actually aren't that busy at all? One of the oldest excuses in the book is, "I don't have enough time." When I hear someone say this, I remind them that even the president of the United States (President Obama at the time of writing this piece), makes time to exercise, to play some basketball, to walk the dog, and to eat dinner with his family! You will always make time for the things you want to do and for the people you value.

The most successful people I've met all have structure and routines to their days. They get up at a certain time, go to the gym at a certain time, eat lunch at the same time, and have set bedtimes. These high achievers have a game plan to their day. They have priorities and tasks that need to be completed by the day's end.

Having a daily written-out, "GET IT DONE!" list makes me more productive. Each night, I'll write down 5 things I need to achieve for the next day. Instead of leaving them for later in the day, I'll usually attempt to do the least favorite tasks first.

Much of life's success comes down to a few key concepts, such as discipline, focus, standards, determination, and consistency. The people who do a good job are those who tend to be more self-reflective and self-aware. With that in mind, I will often monitor a day and see where and how I spend my time.

What matters most is that you take care of the 86,400 seconds in a day to the best of your ability. Whatever you are doing, make that moment count. If you are resting, then shut down completely. If you are training or working, then give your best effort.

* * *

*We all get the same amount of time in a day: 86,400 seconds. The difference is in how we choose to spend that time.*

# The Other Twenty

*Champion minded athletes
are dedicated to a champion lifestyle.*

As a performance and mindset coach, it's always been easy for me to see an athlete's seriousness about improving. I merely needed to observe their lifestyle and habits away from practice time. Elite athletes don't reach the top tiers of their sports through part-time dedication. Reaching the elite level requires a full-time commitment to excellence in every aspect of life.

The average elite athlete spends around 4 hours per day practicing and training. *The other twenty* refers to the other hours in the athlete's day. Champion minded athletes devote themselves to a lifestyle that supports skill development and peak performance. The champion lifestyle includes bedtime and wake time, naps, nutrition, hydration, stretching, journaling, etc. - it all matters. Champion minded athletes realize how they spend the other twenty hours of the day away from practice, contributes to the quality of practice, training, and competition. Those twenty hours represent a substantial amount of time, which directly affects the few hours devoted to training.

Athletes - you rely on coaches and trainers to manage regularly scheduled session hours, but for the other twenty, you are self-reliant. Champion minded athletes are responsible and accountable time managers. They are dedicated to a champion lifestyle, understanding what they do outside of practice contributes massively to their overall success. Those who aspire to be great are the ones who take better care of *the other twenty* hours of the day.

\* \* \*

*Reaching the top in sport is a full-time commitment to a disciplined lifestyle. What you do away from practice time counts just as much as what you during practice.*

*Your effort level is a direct reflection of your interest level.*

*You don't need to tell everyone how invested you are, your actions will do that.*

# The 5 E's of Champion Minded Teammates

*Champion minded athletes and teams have the 5 E's.*

1. They have an irresistible **ENERGY**.

2. They **ELEVATE** their teammates.

3. They always give their best **EFFORT**.

4. They aim for **EXCELLENCE** in their standards.

5. They **ENJOY** competing and the fight.

*When you skip a few reps or cut a corner, you aren't only tricking your coach - you're cheating your teammates and yourself.*

# Confident or Cocky?

*Real confidence comes from within.*

Champion minded athletes know true self-confidence comes from within. They are realistic about their skills and their abilities and how they respond to life's obstacles. They are authentic. They learn from mistakes and their losses do not define them. Instead, they become wiser through their failures and they are stronger and more confident as a result. A person who is truly self-confident is free to be genuinely interested in other people without feeling threatened or inferior. They listen attentively and ask sincere questions.

Cocky people have a false sense of self-worth. They need to be the center of attention, and even if it means putting others down to elevate themselves, they need outside validation.

Confident people are high achievers and through helping others they enjoy contributing to the greater good. They are not threatened by the success of others. Instead, they cheer others on and the learn from the successes and experiences of others.

Cocky people tend to project exaggerated lists of achievements, which are not necessarily realistic. They tend to deny or to belittle the successes of others.

Confident people like to self-reflect, acknowledging their flaws and shortcomings. By being true to themselves, they allow themselves to be vulnerable. When they are wrong, they take ownership of their words and actions.

Cocky people are unwilling to risk looking weak or incompetent. Instead of admitting mistakes, they ignore their flaws and place blame on others.

Confident people don't need to compare themselves to others. Cocky people need to be (or appear to be) better than others. Cocky people are insecure and feel threatened by the prospect of someone else doing better than they are doing.

A champion minded and truly self-confident person doesn't worry about what others think of them. They accept themselves as they are. They are humble and kind, and they stay true to themselves.

\* \* \*

*True self-confidence comes from a very authentic place, a very whole place.*

*Having the skills is only the entry ticket. You need to consistently bring the right attitude, mindset, and work ethic day in and day out.*

# What's Cool and What's Not

*Champion minded athletes have a clear idea of what is cool.*

## Not Cool:

- Arriving late to practice
- Talking while the coach is speaking to the group
- Cutting corners, stopping short of lines, cheating on repetition counts
- Skipping warm-ups and cool-downs, or performing them poorly
- Lack of effort
- Not stretching/neglecting recovery routines
- Eating poorly and not hydrating properly
- Lack of intensity and effort when a coach is not present
- Hanging around with people who distract or poorly influence you
- Quitting/giving up

## Cool:

- Respecting your parents, coaches, and teachers
- Arriving to practice before start time
- Asking for help and advice

- Working hard when the odds are against you
- Outworking the rest
- Working hard with a great attitude
- Taking care of your nutrition and hydration
- Getting enough sleep for proper recovery
- Showing gratitude to those who have helped you
- Trying your hardest and never giving up

# Nadia Comaneci: Champion Minded

*Champion minded athletes do more than what is asked of them.*

Nadia Comaneci is one of my all-time favorite athletes. Nadia was a Romanian gymnast, who at age 14, during the 1976 Summer Olympic Games in Montreal, became the first gymnast in Olympic history to score a perfect 10. I recently watched an interview with Nadia during which she discussed her training routines and her upbringing in then-Communist Romania. When asked if she was pushed too hard by her coaches Bela and Marta Karolyi, she answered,

> *No, I didn't feel that, I actually did a lot more than they were asking me to do and I think about, you know, when coach Bela used to say, 'today we do five routines on beam' and I used to do seven so I could do more than he was asking. I don't mind working hard and don't complain if I work hard. I think that you have to work hard to be up to that level. I think I am not looking for the easy way to do things and I am proud about that. In fact, I was always seeing it as a challenge.*

This is a champion mindset at work. Champion minded athletes choose to go above and beyond what is asked and expected of them. They are intrinsically motivated and driven to succeed. Success is not an accident. It's the result of many years of embracing the grind, rising to challenges, and pushing individual limits. Champions do it for themselves.

Nadia Comaneci did not score a perfect 10 by luck or by chance. Putting in the extra effort to do more than she was asked, she *earned* that score. Nadia represents a great example of a champion minded athlete.

* * *

*Champion minded athletes do more, give more, and achieve more.*

# Skill Acquisition: No Journey is the Same

*Avoid comparing your development with other athletes' development.*

Skill acquisition is made up of three distinct stages - the cognitive stage, the associative stage, and the autonomous stage. As they relate to an athlete's ability to perform a skill or an activity, each stage has its own characteristics. These stages are unique to each athlete's development. Factors include: how often an athlete practices, the types of practice an athlete is engaged in, how an athlete receives and responds to feedback, training intensity and volume, level of competition, etc.

## The Cognitive Stage

An introduction to a skillset or activity, this stage is marked by errors, clumsiness, uncertainty, doubt, and confusion. Athletes: you're going to make mistakes while learning a new skill! Stick with it. There's a great reward in going from feeling uncoordinated and incompetent to feeling confident and masterful!

## The Associative Stage

Once you understand how to perform a skill, you must be able to repeat it. This stage, as in the cognitive stage, requires feedback and adjustment. Athletes: have an open mind to instruction and correction as you learn a new skill and as you train to repeat the new skill. Ask questions. There is a high level of attention to detail involved in learning a skill completely. This is part of deliberate practice. Remember, effort and a focus on improving performance are more important than immediate results!

## The Autonomous Stage

At this stage the skill happens automatically. Once you understand the skill and can successfully repeat it, challenge yourself to perform the skill repeatedly in pressure situations. Daniel Coyle refers to this type of practice in his book *The Talent Code,* "Deep practice is built on a paradox: struggling in certain targeted ways - operating at the edges of your ability, where you make mistakes - makes you smarter." It's generally believed that if you practice long enough, you'll get better. However, if practice is not purposeful and not challenging, an athlete will not successfully develop in the autonomous stage.

\* \* \*

*Focus on your own path, put in the work, and only compare yourself to the person you were yesterday.*

# Purposeful Practice

*Champion minded athletes focus on quality and purposeful practice.*

B ack in 2014, I was invited to observe the U.S. National Badminton Team practice for the World Junior Championships. I've always had great respect and admiration for this sport. If you're not familiar with badminton, it's an extremely punishing and physically demanding sport. In addition to the athleticism of these highly skilled players, the way the coaches created the manner and purpose for the practices impressed me.

## My takeaways:

- Each exercise or drill was measured, had a goal, and a purpose.

- The energy was intense with minimal down time, keeping up the momentum.

- The coaches gave clear, concise instructions, 1-2 lines (John Wooden-like).

- The focus was on quality and purposeful repetition, not just repetition (big difference!).

- Practice partners rotated often and adapted to various playing styles, speeds, and spins, keeping everyone alert.

- They only counted the good repetitions. This resulted in a higher focus and specific purpose.

I call this purposeful practice. The champion minded understand that there's a big difference between going through the motions of practice and practicing with clearly defined parameters and intent. Just logging the practice hours is not enough. To be great, practice requires intensity and purpose. Purposeful practice hours result in success.

\* \* \*

*It's not how much you practice, but how well you do it. It's what you put into those hours that counts most.*

# Put the Phone Down and Get Focused!

## *Distraction is the enemy of success.*

Today we are faced with so many distractions. The cell phone is the most obvious offender. Recently, I observed a women's volleyball team during a track session at a university in Michigan. Half of them had their earphones in and phones in-hand. This is clear evidence of poor standards and a lack of respect for the coach and teammates. To be 100% focused during practice, put down the phone! Listening to coach's instruction, critique, and praise, even when it's not directed at you, it is still an opportunity to learn. Listening to other teammates' questions and comments presents an opportunity to learn and grow as a team. In fact, for the athletes I coach, one of my standards is that cell phones are put away before practice starts. Champion minded athletes understand that full attention, complete focus, and 100% engagement is required in order to achieve greatness.

## Debunking the claims of needing the phone:

☑ "I need it for the stopwatch." Get a stopwatch or a wristwatch and you won't be tempted to sneak a peek at messages and social media while training.

☑ "I need music to keep me motivated." You don't listen to music when you compete. Practice is the time to work on the mental toughness necessary during competition.

☑ "I need it to take notes." Get a journal/notebook. You may want to look over your notes during competition to help you stay focused.

Being coachable means giving full attention. As they understand that complete focus is part of mental toughness, champion minded athletes try to avoid distractions at all costs. 100% engagement means active interest and involvement, necessary parts of a successful team culture. Not all distractions are within your control. Putting down the phone is easy and controllable. Training your mind to stay focused when there is an interruption, hindrance, disturbance, or interference that is beyond your control, is a skill that will help you succeed.

\* \* \*

*Achieving excellence requires being 100% focused and eliminating distractions.*

# Mindset:
# Growth vs Fixed

*Champion minded athletes have
a growth mindset.*

In her book, *Mindset: The New Psychology of Success*, Carol Dweck explores the relationship between an individual's achievement and where they believe ability originates. Individuals who believe success is based on natural ability are said to have a "fixed" mindset. Individuals who believe success is achieved through hard work, continual learning, purposeful training, and resilience are said to have a "growth" mindset. Individuals may not necessarily be aware of their personal mindset, but mindset reveals itself in their reaction to failure. Fixed mindset individuals fear failure, because they view it as a factor which negatively defines their capability. Growth mindset individuals do not fear failure because they perceive failure to be an opportunity to learn and improve. In a 2012 interview, Dweck defines fixed and growth mindsets as such:

> *In a fixed mindset, students believe their basic abilities, their intelligence, their talents, are just fixed traits. They have a certain amount and that's that, and then their goal becomes to look smart all the time and never look dumb. In a growth mindset, students understand that their talents and abilities can be developed through effort,*

*good teaching, and persistence. They don't necessarily think everyone's the same or anyone can be Einstein, but they believe everyone can get smarter if they work at it.*

Champion minded athletes have a growth mindset and are more likely to continue working hard despite setbacks. They welcome criticism and embrace challenges. A fixed minded athlete is oversensitive to criticism, avoids challenges, and gives up easily for fear of "looking bad." Growth minded athletes take responsibility and are accountable for their development. Fixed mindset athletes make excuses and place blame. Growth minded athletes are coachable, they listen to advice and they are open to making changes. Fixed minded athletes are skeptical, they don't listen, they become defensive, they are closed minded, and reluctant to change. Sadly, fixed minded athletes rarely reach their full potential.

\* \* \*

*A champion minded athlete has a growth mindset. They see obstacles and challenges as great opportunities to learn and improve.*

*Fixed mindset athletes have a defeatist attitude, whereas growth mindset athletes persist in the face of adversity.*

# Get Comfortable Being Uncomfortable

*When you're cruising, you're losing.*

Champion minded athletes know that a comfort zone is a no-progress zone. If you are just cruising along, you'll soon be left behind. Staying comfortable means being complacent. Complacency is self-satisfaction while unaware of deficiencies. Comfort zones are home to the apathetic, the perfunctory, the dispassionate.

Getting out of your comfort zone requires honest self-reflection. Are your habits helping you reach your goals? Are the people you surround yourself with encouraging you, challenging you, and helping you to reach your goals? Are you challenging yourself or are you playing it safe? Champion minded athletes push themselves to succeed by getting out of their comfort zones and embracing the struggle, knowing that often things get worse before they get better. Many athletes get comfortable where they are and avoid change, but there can be no progress without change. Get comfortable being uncomfortable. Do more of what challenges you everyday. Remember, that all progress takes place outside your comfort zone.

\* \* \*

*"I like to push myself during practice. I have always been about getting uncomfortable, because that's where we grow most."*

- Paige Williams, English professional football player

# There Are No Shortcuts To The Top

*Champion minded athletes ask more of themselves.*

There are no shortcuts to the top. There's no way around the grind. You get what you give. Champion minded athletes do more than what is asked of them. They ask more of themselves.

Regardless of who is watching, champion minded athletes are consistent in their effort and work ethic. Doing what you are supposed to do when coaches, trainers, parents, and teammates are around is one thing, but what you do when no one is watching is quite another. Maybe you adhere to others' standards when you have to, but your own personal standards are what reveal your true commitment. Do you do your homework only when pushed by a parent or coach? Do you do just enough to get by? Or are you pushing yourself, asking more of yourself, and testing your own limits? Athletes: by cutting corners, you are only cheating yourself. If your effort depends on who is watching, meaning you work hard when a parent or a coach is present, but slack off when they aren't there, you are hurting your chances to achieve your goals. It all matters - the effort you give when no one is watching, directly impacts your long-term success.

Legendary basketball player, Michael Jordan once said, "There are no shortcuts. I approached practices the same way I approached games. You can't turn it on and off like a faucet, I couldn't dog it during practice and then when I needed that extra push late in the game, expect it to be there. Very few people get anywhere by taking shortcuts."

At the highest levels of sport, success is in the smallest details. When I asked 6x Olympian and 4x gold medalist in Ice Hockey, Hayley Wickenheiser, what she saw in the very best players, she said: "The best are consistent in the day-to-day things. They have world-class work ethics and standards."

When you reach an elite level, everyone is good at what they do. So often, the smallest of margins - an inch, a millisecond, a hundredth of a point, a buzzer beater - creates the win. Champion minded athletes are detail oriented. They push themselves and they don't cut corners.

\* \* \*

*"Very few people get anywhere by taking shortcuts."*

\- Michael Jordan

# Comparison is a No-Win Game!

*Champion minded athletes do not compare their progress with others.*

One of the main reasons we are discontent with our lives is because we are always comparing ourselves with others. We measure how well we are doing in comparison with others. We make mistakes or don't make quick enough progress and therefore we feel inferior. We experience success and progress and we begin to feel superior. Our confidence and our self-belief moves with the market and flows with the opinions of others.

In life, comparing yourself to others will always be a losing game. Like it or not, there will always be someone smarter, faster, stronger, more wealthy, more attractive, or more talented than you are. But here is what they don't have - the amazing abundance of uniqueness and talents you have! There is no one quite like you. If you're so busy comparing your life or yourself to what others have or do, it leaves you with less time and energy to bring out the best in you. The best person you can compare yourself to is the person you were yesterday - just try and improve on that!

When it comes to sports, comparing yourself with others can be unproductive and a waste of energy. It's especially prevalent regarding progress and results. The fact that each athlete has a unique genetic code, culture, upbringing, and support system renders comparison unsubstantial. Each athlete is on their own unique journey, making it unrealistic and unreasonable to compare one person's progress with that of another. Each athlete progresses and develops at a different rate.

Athletes - avoid the temptation to compare your development and your results with others. Stay focused on your own goals and path. When it comes to comparison, focus on comparing yourself to the person you were yesterday.

* * *

*It takes persistence, patience, and time to reach worthwhile long-term goals.*

# What to Say When You Talk to Yourself

*Champion minded athletes are serial self-talkers.*

I'll admit it - I talk to myself pretty much all day. It's something I've been working on for years. I've learned that no matter how many positive things I might hear and read, I still need to take control of the voice in my head.

A positive attitude and a strong, supportive inner voice require consistent and purposeful practice – lots of it. In others words, just like your game skills, it requires daily work.

In sports, we see athletes start their events in a positive frame of mind, radiating great body language, and walking with marked confidence. However, the moment difficulty or fatigue arises, a few errors begin to creep in and we see those positive traits begin to transform. The positive thoughts and self-talk have disappeared. Doubt, frustration, negativity, and fear have replaced taken hold.

How you talk to yourself is critical. Self-talk manifests itself in your beliefs, your words, and your actions. If you listen to your subconscious mind, you'll hear lots of noise about doubt and fear. Choose to talk to yourself instead of listening to yourself. This one simple adjustment can change everything. During competition when things don't go according to plan (it's inevitable), you need to self-coach and self-motivate in your own mind.

Improving your self-talk requires a daily effort - at home, at work, at school, on the sports field, etc. It's a habit developed through consistent practice. Through this habit, we conquer the inner voice that shouts complaints, self-doubt, fear, and negativity - all of which lead to unhappiness and a lesser performance. Positive people can have negative thoughts. The difference lies in how quickly they can let go of those thoughts and focus on the positive.

Athletes: how often are you consciously working on your self-talk on the practice court or the field? Like your game skills, your mindset needs much attention. If you don't purposely work on it, you can't get better at it. If you were to rate yourself from 1-10 regarding your self-talk under pressure or when playing below your expected level, what would it be?

* * *

*Positive people can have negative thoughts.*
*The difference lies in how quickly they can let go of*
*those negative thoughts and focus on the positive.*

# Feedback

*Ask for feedback, accept it, and apply it!*

Champion minded athletes crave feedback. They are open to criticism. They believe the only way they are going to progress is to receive feedback from their coaches and their team. They don't get defensive or take it personally. Instead, they hear it for what it is - an invitation and encouragement to improve.

Being coachable involves being open to feedback and criticism. Craving feedback is a common trait amongst the very best athletes in the world. NBA Basketball All Star player Stephen Curry once said, "I need coaches who can tell me what I am doing wrong so I can get better." Former England and Liverpool soccer captain, Steven Gerrard, once said, "Feedback is crucial if you want to become your best. Being open to receiving it is what helps you improve." These athletes epitomize coach-ability.

Athletes who are not open to feedback close the door on the opportunity to improve themselves. If you can't accept someone telling you what you need to hear, it's impossible to get better. In many cases, inflated egos have been the enemy of many athletes who wanted to progress in their careers. In other cases athletes are unwilling to make a change that will lower performance level in the short-term before raising performance level in the long-term.

How well do you receive criticism and feedback? How then, do you go about making changes based on that feedback? Understand that how well you accept and apply feedback will determine your level of success. Don't let an ego or fear of change or a short-term dip in results get in the way of your progress.

An openness to learning is another factor distinguishing the good from the great. As an athlete, if you aren't open to criticism and receiving feedback, then you aren't serious about getting better.

* * *

*A champion minded athlete craves feedback.*
*They always want to know what they can do better.*

# Discipline

*Discipline drives high performance results.*

If there is one thing I've learned about discipline over the years, it's this: the average minded hate it, but the champion minded love it.

The more discipline you have, the more freedom you gain. Discipline brings reward. The more disciplined you are and the longer you commit to it, the greater the rewards become. Discipline gives you choice. It puts you in a position of advantage, not entitlement.

Discipline is different than motivation. Motivation can be fleeting. Discipline is a constant choice that you develop over time. It's about doing what you should do even when you don't feel like doing it, and doing it with effort and a good attitude.

Champion minded athletes view discipline as one of the main keys to being world-class. No champion performer or team has reached the top without discipline. Discipline is not punishment. It is necessary to achieve excellence. It's what drives high performance results.

\* \* \*

*Discipline: the average hate it, the champion minded love it.*

*The champion minded realize that reaching an elite level in a sport first requires a professional approach to their daily habits and lifestyle.*

# SECTION 3:

# *Developmental Training*

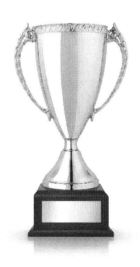

# 10 Core Standards

## *Champion minded athletes have a fundamental set of standards.*

1. Start by having a game plan and a structure to each day.

2. Keep a journal and a record each day.

3. Schedule your bedtime and wake up time to ensure the proper amount of sleep.

4. Eat a healthy, balanced breakfast (I recommend oatmeal, fruit, and 15-25g protein).

5. Designate daily recovery time (I recommend stretching and foam rolling 10 minutes in the morning and 10 minutes in the evening).

6. Spend 20 minutes each day reading motivational/inspirational/ spiritual material (I recommend doing this at the start of each day to shape your daily mindset).

7. Stay hydrated. Keep water with you, and sip throughout the day.

8. Plan and pack healthy snacks to eat throughout the day

9. Schedule a daily nap.

10. Maintain your own equipment, and pack your bag the night before.

\* \* \*

*"Without self-discipline, success is impossible, period."*

\- Lou Holtz

# Pre-Breakfast Productivity

## *Champion minded athletes get a great head start on their day.*

The most important and productive hours of my day come before breakfast. Champion minded athletes choose the lifestyle habit of getting up early and following a productive routine. They know that the most important time of the day is before other people are even awake!

Over time, I have built effective routines and habits into my lifestyle. These habits put me in a champion frame of mind. My routine helps me feel ready to face whatever the day may bring, and to do so with good energy and a positive mindset. Achieving greatness in little ways adds up to achieving greatness in big ways.

All too often, I hear people use the excuse that "they don't have time." We all have the time, it just takes getting up a little earlier in the day. What I love most about this time is that it is exclusively MY time.

It's important to make time for yourself to live a happy, healthy life.

## My personal morning routine is as follows:

- 20 minutes reading motivational or spiritual passages
- 20 minutes stretching and foam rolling
- 20 minutes checking/posting on my twitter (yes, it's important)
- 20 minutes practicing thoughtfulness and gratitude

M

*Champion minded athletes
have set morning routines.*

# Ante Meridiem (a.m.)

*Have an attitude management check
every morning.*

We know that time listed as "a.m." refers to the morning; "a.m." is the abbreviation of the Latin *ante meridiem*, which means "before noon." For our purpose relating to champion minded athletes, "a.m." stands for "attitude management." When starting your day, the attitude you choose is crucial for determining how the rest of your day unfolds. That is why it's so important for you to choose a great start!

I often hear, "But Allistair, I'm just not a morning person." I understand that not everyone naturally wakes up bright and cheery, but I believe you are not *born* a morning or an evening person, you are *made* a morning person or evening person. You condition yourself through your habits, which develop over time. In other words, you train your mind and body to be a certain way.

I have never met a successful person who sleeps in on a regular basis. Sure, occasionally sleeping in is ok and maybe even some extra rest is necessary; but making it a habit will only impede your success. Champion minded athletes are early risers who are eager to start the day. Go tell a Michael Phelps, Tom Brady, or Kerry Walsh that you're not a morning person, and they will tell you that you just aren't fully committed to reaching the top. Champion minded performers have trained themselves to be morning people. They are driven. They consistently choose to start the day early with a positive attitude and a desire to work hard.

Labeling yourself as "not a morning person" may be an indication that it's time to change some of your habits (specifically your bedtime). When you find yourself feeling grouchy or unmotivated, then it's time to pause, and to have a little attitude management (a.m.) check with yourself.

Remember, starting your day properly is vital to your success. In order to start your day champion minded, add an attitude management check to your morning routine.

\* \* \*

*Biggest precursor of success? The attitude you choose on a daily basis.*

*Attitude is a skill that needs to be trained every single day.*

# Ask Yourself This Question Every Morning

*"How can I get better today?"*

The champion minded are on a mission to improve themselves and those around them. Each morning they wake up and ask themselves one simple question: "How can I get better today?"

Everyday is a new day to get a little bit better, an opportunity to improve on the day before, to get one step closer to the vision and goal. The champion minded know yesterday is the past and today is what matters most. As they progress toward their vision, they understand what they do on a daily basis matters most.

Each day you need to have a game plan and a structure to your day. Without one, you are letting the day run you instead of you running the day. Having no plan nor structure to your day is like a pilot having no direction nor flight plan for his flight. He's going to be flying aimlessly.

Opportunity is everywhere. In life, there are too many people just happy to get by. I believe that if you work hard and have a greater purpose, you will succeed. It's easy to live life on cruise control, to do what you've always done. When you are cruising, you're losing. When you are comfortably in cruise control, those others putting in the extra work are passing you by.

How are you starting your day? Are you challenging yourself to get better or are you just hoping things will miraculously happen?

Do your daily standards challenge you, or do they allow you to just get by? Talent is a gift. Hard work is a choice. Remember, there is no middle ground. Each day you are either getting better or you are getting left behind.

The champion minded wake up every morning and ask themselves, "How can I get better today?" They have a structure and a game plan for their day. From there, they attack the day with determination and purpose!

* * *

*Each morning on waking,*
*the champion minded ask themselves,*
*"How can I get better today?"*

*Getting better is about competing against yourself.*
*It's about self- improvement and aiming to be better than you were the day before.*

# Structure Your Day

*Champion minded athletes*
*live structured days with clear direction.*

To achieve greatness in any area of your life you need to have structure to your day. Developing daily routines is a crucial element to organization and productivity. Former U.S. Secretary of State, Colin Powell, gave a TED talk on kids and why they need structure. In his talk, Powell explains that providing kids with structure is not about limiting freedom, but about providing a solid foundation to build their future. He says that without structure, people waste time and energy on indecisiveness, idleness, incompetence, and inefficiency.

To be structured is to be organized according to a plan of action for a specific purpose. A few years ago, a professional athlete asked me to come to New York and to help him prepare for the upcoming World Championships. I had not worked with him prior to this opportunity, and I quickly realized the main hindrance to his progress had nothing to do with his training. He lacked structure in his day. His wake up times and bed times were inconsistent and his nutritional habits were erratic. Instead of being in control of his days, his days were in control of him. Before we could go forward with a training program, we had to develop daily routines to create a structure in which we could effectively and efficiently work.

Success starts by having structure and routines built into your day. Successful athletes and teams require a structural foundation. Adding structure to your day improves sports performance and improves your life. Champion minded athletes have structure and a game plan to their day. They understand this will conserve vital energy and build winning systems.

## 5 benefits of having structure to your day:

1. Provides a game plan

2. Saves energy

3. Increases productivity

4. Improves time management and organization

5. Identifies priorities

\* \* \*


*As an athlete, you need structure to your day,
a game plan to follow.*

# Hydrate All Day

## *Hydration is an all-day habit.*

Driving a car without water eventually burns up the engine. Just as cars require regular maintenance to function properly, our bodies require regular care to function properly.

Having spent a great deal of time observing athletes and their habits, I've discovered that even though they might be excellent at putting in the hard yards at the gym, on the court, or on the field, they still fall terribly short in the hydration department.

Here in the heat of Florida, I recently performed a hydration test on a British athlete, to see how much liquid he would need to stay hydrated during a two-hour practice. In those two hours, this 165 lbs male athlete had lost a staggering 9 lbs - just through sweat loss! Athletes who lose more than 2 percent of their body weight, (3 pounds for a 150-pound athlete) lose both their mental edge and their ability to perform optimally.

Hydration must be an all-day habit. Only drinking before and during practice is not good enough for the athlete. Waiting until you are thirsty is too late. You're already dehydrated. Did you know that you are already in a dehydrated state when you wake up in the morning? That's why it's a great habit to have a glass of water upon waking each morning and to always keep water next to your bed.

For better performance and recovery, sip water throughout the day. Leave water bottles around the house, office, in the car, or wherever you might be. This helps remind you that you need to keep sipping.

* * *

*For the athlete, staying hydrated must be an all-day habit.*

# Daytime Naps

*Champion minded athletes*
*make daily nap time a priority.*

As a performance and mindset coach, one of my goals is to do everything I can (within the rules) to maximize an athlete's performance. Obtaining high performance in sports isn't only about what takes place in the gym or on the field. Often, what happens away from the training area matters more. So, I need to know details regarding each individual athlete's equipment, nutrition/hydration, training schedule, daily habits, competitive schedule, academic schedule, physical/mental/emotional status, and social engagements. Every aspect contributes to optimal performance training.

A crucial part of maximizing performance is setting aside time in the day for a nap. Napping for 20-30 minutes is recognized as a key factor to athletic performance. Professional football (soccer) programs such as Real Madrid and Bayern Munich, as well as American Universities such as Oregon and Clemson, include nap rooms in their training centers. Recently, when talking with the LA Lakers performance coach, Tim DeFrancisco, he mentioned their players regularly take a nap before practice or competition. NBA professionals LeBron James and Stephen Curry also schedule daytime naps. Dan McCarthy, USA National Swim Team's high performance consultant, advocates the benefits of daily naps. Athletes - if you want to improve your performance, include a short nap into your daily routine.

On training days and on recovery days, Grand Slam champion and Olympic Gold Medalist, Andy Murray makes his daily nap a priority. Whether you are working in a split schedule of two training sessions in a day, training before and/or after school, in order to maximize the practice session, it is important to schedule a short nap.

Champion minded athletes take naps and come to practice more rested, alert, and ready to train. Athletes who take naps are more productive, have less risk of injury, absorb and process information more easily - all of which lead to better long-term results.

* * *

*"If you get a nap in everyday, all those hours add up and it allows you to get through the season better."*

- Steve Nash

# Recovery

*Champion minded athletes train and recover like champions.*

When I was a professional athlete, I didn't respect recovery enough. It probably cost me a few wins and a few extra years on my athletic career. Only later did I realize athletic success relies on more than hard work. Recovery is just as critical a component to athletic achievement. Champion minded athletes understand the importance of proper regeneration and recovery for their bodies and minds.

It is no secret among athletes that in order to improve performance you've got to work hard. However, after the hard work, it's the rest that makes you stronger. During recovery periods, your energy and muscular systems are able to restore and to rebuild, to recover from the stress they endured during training. The result is a higher level of performance. If sufficient rest is not scheduled into the training program, then regeneration cannot occur and performance will suffer. If this imbalance between a higher workload and inadequate rest persists, then performance will decline and the risk of injury increases.

Overtraining can be defined as the state where the athlete has been repeatedly stressed by training to the point where rest is no longer adequate to allow for recovery. Overtraining can cause problems like reduced performance, poor sleep, increased injury risk, and slower recovery from competition. It can also lead to longer-term issues such as chronic fatigue. To make continual improvements, athletes require adequate recovery and regeneration to allow their bodies to adjust to the increases in workload and to help avoid long term fatigue and chronic injuries.

The champion minded athlete recognizes rest and recovery are a vital part of training. Being aware of how you feel physically, mentally, and emotionally impacts performance. Keeping track of general health, muscle soreness, fatigue, and mood is significant and helpful in signaling overtraining. When early signs of overtraining are present, athletes should adjust the work-to-rest ratio and the schedule to allow for recovery. Champion minded athletes are in tune with their health and they are aware of the warning signs of overtraining.

\* \* \*

*"You don't get strong by just working hard, you get strong by resting after having worked hard."*

- Ned Overend

# The Importance of Sleep

*Champion minded athletes prioritize sleep.*

Sleep is a major contributor to peak athletic performance. Sleep affects moods, energy, focus, and concentration. Champion minded athletes adhere to the highest standards regarding their physical conditioning, nutrition, hydration, and overall preparation in order to achieve peak performance. These include the quality and amount of sleep.

Much is said about diet and exercise programs, but sleep is rarely part of the conversation. To ignore the importance of sleep is to disregard a critical aspect of performance and recovery. Athletes: the quality and quantity of sleep can be a distinguishing factor between who performs well or poorly on game-day. Getting the right amount of good quality sleep can bring more consistent performance, quicker recovery, better motivation, and clearer decision-making.

Having a scheduled bedtime and wake time is critical to achieving greatness in sport and in life. Thinking about when you go to bed at night and when you wake in the morning are the first steps to reaching your potential. Athletes: because you regularly train, travel, and compete, you need more sleep than average people. Training, traveling, and competing places your mind, body, and spirit under more stress. Consequently, you require more sleep to recover and to do it all again.

Lack of sleep literally slows you down - it reduces your reaction time. Lack of sleep also deprives the body of the time needed for regeneration, which weakens the immune system and increases the risk of injury or illness. Well-rested athletes are stronger, healthier, faster, more accurate, and they use better judgement in decision-making.

I always remind the athletes I work with - if you aren't getting the right amount of sleep every night, then you aren't serious about being the best you can be! Sleep is the foundation of all performance - it all starts there!

* * *

*Peak performance requires the proper amount of good quality sleep.*

# World-class athletes who make sleep a top priority:

- **Usain Bolt** (8-time Olympic gold medalist, 11-time World Champion): 8-10 hours

- **Roger Federer** (18-time Grand Slam Champion, Davis Cup Champion, Olympic gold medalist): 10-12 hours

- **LeBron James** (3-time NBA Champion, 4-time NBA MVP, 2-time Olympic gold medalist): 12 hours

- **Rory McIlroy** (Major Golf champion): 9 hours

- **Andy Murray** (3-time Grand Slam Champion, 2-time Olympic medalist, Davis Cup Champion): 11-12 hours

- **Rafael Nadal** (14-time Grand Slam Champion, Olympic gold medalist, 4-time Davis Cup Champion): 8-9 hours

- **Michael Phelps** (28 Olympic medals): 9-10 hours

- **Sebastian Vettel** (4-time Formula One World Champion): 8-9 hours

- **Lindsay Vonn** (4-time World Cup Champion, 5-time World Championship medalist, Olympic gold medalist): 9-10 hours

- **Russell Wilson** (NFL winning quarterback for the Seattle Seahawks): 7-8 hours

# Mini-Regeneration Zones

*Champion minded athletes
have designated mini-regeneration zones.*

I was recently watching a documentary on Cristiano Ronaldo, the Real Madrid and Portuguese soccer star. One segment led viewers on a tour of Ronaldo's impressive home located in the outer suburbs of Madrid. Of all the stunning aspects of Ronaldo's house, his home gym and training facility impressed me the most. It had everything to keep one of the world's best soccer players in peak condition. The space designated for recovery and regeneration especially amazed me. Included in his home training facility, was a hot/cold tub for recovery, a cryotherapy tank, and various other pieces of recovery equipment.

The consummate professional, Ronaldo not only understands the importance of training hard, but also of recovering well. If you haven't recovered from your previous work, your body cannot push or perform to the optimum level. The champion minded athlete understands that to perform at the highest level, they need to consistently be taking care of their body and their recovery efforts.

Understandably, we all don't have the budget or the luxury of having a facility in our homes like Ronaldo does, but we can still have the same mindset and approach when it comes to the importance of recovery. Just having a few regeneration tools at home is already a step in the right direction. I advise my athletes to have a *mini-regeneration zone* at home. A mini-regeneration zone is an area in your living space devoted to recovery. Some examples of recovery tools to include in your mini-regeneration zone are: a stretch strap, a foam roller, and a trigger ball. These recovery tools are easily transportable, and I recommend setting up a mini-regeneration zone in your hotel room when traveling. Instead of keeping them packed away in your bag, designate an area and set out your recovery tools so they are visible.

Whether with their teammates during set practice time, or on their own time, by performing these mini routines, the champion minded athlete is always taking care of his or her body. In addition to what you do with your team and your coach, I recommend performing at least 20 minutes of regeneration daily. Champion minded athletes know that consistently taking care of their health and wellness (and staying injury-free) are critical components to peak performance.

*  *  *

*The key to world-class performance lies in how well you recover after working hard.*

# Travel & Nutrition

*Champion minded athletes
come prepared ahead of time.*

I have always believed that you can tell the difference between the players who are serious about getting better and those who only talk about it. Those who want to get better show it in their actions and prepare a little bit extra. When it comes to nutrition and travel, I always think back to this story:

It was early January and I was sitting in the waiting lounge at the Sarasota/Bradenton airport in Florida, getting ready for the start of another tennis season in Australia. There, I bumped into my former next door neighbor, a young Japanese player, who eventually went on to reach the top 5 in the world rankings. It was great to reconnect. As we were chatting, he proceeded to pull out three assortments of foods. In carefully-wrapped bags, he had some grilled chicken, vegetables, and chopped apples. At that moment, I realized just how serious he was about achieving his goals and how determined he was to be one of the best players in the world (at the time he had just broken into the top 50). I asked him who had prepared his food, and he looked at me a bit surprised and said, "I did, of course." It would have been much easier to just buy some food at the airport or on the airplane.

These are the small things that the very best are committed to doing and something I try to instill in every athlete I train. They are choices. Do you think he found it fun to cook and to prepare his own travel food? I doubt it. But, he was willing to do what it took to reach the top. It comes down to choice and effort.

Champion minded athletes don't take a chance on whether or not the airport will have what they need. They prepare ahead of time and avoid the stress or panic if what they need is not available. They make the efforts and know they will pay off in the longer term.

* * *

*Champion minded athletes plan and prepare ahead of time when it comes to their nutrition and traveling.*

*Everyone's good when things are good. It's the moment fatigue and pressure set in that exposes who has developed the right mindset and habits, and who hasn't.*

# Listening Skills

*Champion minded athletes are great listeners.*

Over the years of coaching, I have recognized a striking quality among the best athletes. I see it especially in the younger athletes who progress more quickly - they are coachable and they are great listeners. These athletes listen with more than their ears - they listen with all of their senses - they watch intently, they listen carefully, they aren't talking, they aren't distracted, they aren't doing something else (bouncing a ball, etc.), their attention is undivided. They absorb information like sponges. They imitate demonstrations. They repeat key words and phrases to themselves. They ask questions and they take it all in.

Champion minded athletes listen with all of their senses and they are respectful of the speaker. They listen intently because they recognize an opportunity to learn and to improve. Listening skills are an important quality in athletics and in life. When you talk, you are only telling someone something you know. But, when you listen, you learn.

Champion minded athletes are coachable, listening to criticism and applying advice in practice to improve. Champion minded athletes seek feedback in order to grow. Champion minded athletes are respectful, maintain eye-contact, and give undivided attention to who is speaking. They don't want to miss an opportunity to learn something new!

\* \* \*

M

*Champion minded athletes*
*don't only listen with their ears,*
*they listen with all of their senses.*

# Communication

*The best teams have
great communication skills.*

How invested are you in your progress? How well do you communicate with your coaches and your support team?

One of my favorite things to do is to learn from other sports. I'm a big fan of Formula One motor racing, a sport similar to American Indy car racing. It's an incredibly technical and detailed sport. The champion drivers aren't the ones who just drive the fastest, but rather, the ones who can provide their teams with the best feedback. They are scholars of their sports.

Many years back, whilst growing up in South Africa, I attended a free practice session for the Rothmans Honda Formula One Team. At the time, their driver was Canadian, Jacque Villeneuve. In practice, Jacque would take the car out for a lap and return to the pits to provide his team of mechanics and technicians with information about how the car was handling and what could be improved. This process carried on the whole day - a lap out on the track followed by 30 or so minutes back in the pits. The team immediately surrounded the car to listen to the feedback and to make the adjustments.

Decathlete and double Olympic gold medalist, Aston Eaton, is great example of someone who invests in their own development. The American athlete was exceptional at providing his coach, Harry Marra, with constant and consistent feedback. Marra stated that Eaton was so invested in continual improvement that he was always willing to honestly and openly share what he was feeling and thinking.

Like a Formula One driver, or Aston Eaton, the champion minded athletes are great at providing feedback. They communicate with their support teams in order to have the best possible preparation for success.

* * *

*Great communication is what makes a team strong.*

# Building Confidence

## *Self-Talk + Preparation + Momentum = Confidence*

"How can I be more confident?" I'm asked this question quite often and my answer is always the same, "Continually improve your self-talk, prepare to your best ability, and keep looking for the positives in every situation." Self-talk is key. You can talk yourself in to or out of just about anything. Being self-critical and always looking for what's wrong only breaks down your confidence and self-belief. Instead, try to focus on affirming yourself when you perform well. You can't stop negative thoughts from entering the mind, but you can control the amount of time you allow those thoughts to stay. Successful self-talk comes from replacing a negative thought with a positive thought.

A huge part of confidence comes from the time you dedicate to your preparation. During each training session, the physical, mental, and emotional work you put in builds confidence. This requires a belief in the process - trusting that your coaches, trainers, teammates, and support system are centered around your needs and have your best interest at heart.

Momentum is a key factor in shaping confidence. Lets face it, if you are continually injured or ill, it's difficult to win. When building confidence, see every win, no matter how big or small, as another building block on the foundation of your confidence.

Lastly, it's important to surround yourself with people who believe in you and encourage you. Avoid those people who are hyper-critical, who discourage you, and who cause you to doubt yourself. Confidence is a skill that requires consistent care.

## 5 Keys to Building Confidence:

1. Practice positive self-talk on a daily basis.

2. Stop the self-critical talk and negative focus.

3. Believe in the process and trust it.

4. Gain momentum through the small wins, they lead to bigger victories!

5. Surround yourself with people that build you up.

* * *

*"Winning breeds confidence and confidence breeds winning."*

- Hubert Green

*Being self-critical and always looking for what's wrong will only break down your confidence and self-belief. Instead, focus on catching yourself doing things right, no matter how small they may seem. Compliment yourself! This is how you build confidence.*

# Body Language:
# Your Unspoken Message

*Your body hears everything your mind says.*

Body language is communication without words. Body language is vital in athletics and in life. Classic signs of poor body language are slumped and drawn-in shoulders, head down, heavy and slowly dragging feet. These physical indicators communicate defeat. We are also familiar with the traditional postures of victory - arms raised or outstretched, shoulders back, face looking toward the sky, maybe leaping with joy. Your body language tells your opponent how you're feeling and what you're thinking. Displaying poor body language gives your opponent extra energy and confidence. Developing positive body language is a trainable skill. Maintaining good posture, keeping your head up and eyes forward, walking tall with confidence, and showing positive energy despite how angry, frustrated, or disappointed you may feel is an importance skill. We can act our way to positive thinking sooner than we can think our way to positive acting.

Sometimes you have to *fake it until you make it*. When you aren't performing at your desired level, it's important to display the same body language that you do when you are performing well. Body language routines are especially beneficial to help with nervousness and anxiety. Consider gymnastics. A gymnast's dismount counts toward their overall score. Even after an extra step, hop, wobble, or fall, they still must stand and display victorious posture. USA gymnast Kerri Strug's vault performance at the 1996 Olympic games is forever imprinted on my mind. To win the gold medal for the team, Kerri had to connect on her vault performance. During her first vault attempt, she fell and injured her left ankle badly. Limping away from the mat, she looked to her coach, Bela Karolyi, and he encouraged her, yelling, "you can do it, you can do it!" She did it. She actually landed the vault on one leg, arms up, shoulders back, eyes to the sky, before collapsing to her knees, face distorted in pain, and having to be carried off the mat by the medical staff and her coach.

If you maintain confident body language during the highest pressure situations, it sends a powerful and clear message to your opponent, teammates, coaches, and/or judges. Champion minded athletes understand that in the pressure filled moments of competition they reveal their habits developed during practice.

I encourage you to work on improving your body language everyday. Just like your game skills, it's something that needs to be practiced.

* * *

*Champion minded athletes*
*display the body language of a champion.*

# No Off Days

*A rest day doesn't mean a "do nothing day."*

If you are serious about becoming your very best, then you have to stay disciplined in the daily routines and pay attention to the details. In elite sport, there are no off days. To the champion minded, every day has a purpose, be it a training day or a rest day. Each day the choices you make contribute to reaching your goals. Depending on how well the athlete has recovered from the previous workload, each individual athlete's training program should include one or two free days per week, however, a free day is not an off day. Free days still include routines within the overall process, such as stretching, foam rolling, massage therapy, nutrition, and hydration. In training, or even in competition, after a complete day off, I have often seen athletes come back worse off. In other words, they did absolutely nothing, were tight, sluggish, and slow.

Stretching and foam rolling routines generate blood flow and help with muscle restoration. Recovery techniques aim to keep muscles long and joints loose. The intensity and quality of your workload during training relates to the time and effort devoted to your recovery. The goal is to be physically and mentally prepared for each new training session or competition by being mindful of workload intensity and the necessary recovery to avoid injury and to stay on the track to success.

Whether it is a work day or a rest day, champion minded athletes continually take care of their bodies and minds. They understand the importance of recovery and the importance of taking care of themselves. Elite sports are about managing the small details that add up to greater success! When striving for excellence, you are responsible for continual attention to your body and mind.

Do the little bits and pieces each day, and take better care of yourself!

\* \* \*

*It's not rocket science that the better you recover, the better you perform.*

# Solo Time

*Champion minded athletes*
*spend time working on their skills alone.*

op athletes put in a tremendous amount of work on their own time. They are consistently driven to do more, to work harder, and they are willing to put in the extra practice hours by themselves. In addition to his training with a coach or practice partner, squash World Champion and former World Number 1, Ramy Ashour, devoted hours upon hours to solo practice. Regarded as one of the most skilled athletes to play the game, his relentless efforts led him to achieve success. He wasn't just gifted with natural talent. During his structured, coach-led practices, as well as his solo training, he earned his way to elite status through diligent work.

Dan Carter, rugby union player for New Zealand's national team, the All Blacks, was known to spend hours alone, honing his kicking skills after the team practice had ended. Considered by many to be the greatest ice hockey player of all time, Wayne Gretzky denies innate abilities. He explains that his development derived from his extraordinary commitment to time on the ice. In his autobiography he wrote, "All I wanted to do in the winters was be on the ice. I'd get up in the morning, skate from 7:00-8:30, go to school, come home at 3:30, stay on the ice until my mom insisted I come in for dinner, eat in my skates, then go back out until 9:00." In cooperation with his coaches, Gretzky attributes his hockey instincts and skills to his tireless efforts to study and to practice the game.

Cara Black was once the number one doubles tennis player in the world. Growing up, Cara would spend endless hours hitting against a wall outside her home, working on her volleying skills. There's even a great YouTube video of her performing 100 close range volleys against the wall at lightning speed.

Champion minded athletes are driven to do extra work on their own time. They spend time practicing solo. They know that success is never by accident. It is the result of a great desire and a willingness to work harder than the rest.

How much extra time are you putting in?

\* \* \*

*"Success is born out of faith, an undying passion, and a relentless drive."*

- Stephen Curry

# Know When to Fold 'em

*Champion minded athletes*
*always aim to finish practice on a positive.*

A s a coach, one of my goals is to make sure that we always finish practice on a positive note. No matter how good or bad the practice may have gone that day, the goal is to finish on a high.

How you feel when you leave practice often stays with you until the next session. By finishing practice on a positive note, you take with you a feeling of achievement and positive energy, characteristics which ultimately build confidence.

Another important factor to a successful practice is knowing when it's quitting time. Many times I will witness players feeling they need to "fill the time." If you've booked the court or pitch for two hours, then don't feel the need to use all of the two hours. There's no need to be a slave to the clock during practice. If you have achieved your main focus for practice before the time is up, it's ok to finish practice early. That doesn't mean you're lazy or taking the easier route. Often I will hear, "But Allistair, you always say that we should do more if we want to become champion minded!" This is true, but sometimes you just need to be satisfied with the work you've put in for that day.

If you are trying a certain task and becoming increasingly frustrated, it's ok to put it aside and to try again another day. Go back to a familiar game that will be fun and which will allow you to leave practice with a feeling of accomplishment. Finish on a positive! The memory of that last beautiful swing, throw, serve, catch, kick, or play will have a lasting impression and will build confidence for the next session.

\* \* \*

*Practice is a little bit like gambling. In order to win, you need to learn to quit while you're ahead.*

# Progress Takes Time

*Champion minded athletes stay patient,*
*but never complacent.*

P rogress isn't always easily measured, especially on a daily basis. So often, athletes are impatient - they want to see results now! They desire instant gratification instead of patiently trusting the process. Champion minded athletes know that progress takes time. They invest in the long term journey.

Developing the skills to be successful in a certain field takes years and years of hard work, purposeful repetition, and a mindset committed to the process. For elite professionals there is no such thing as an overnight success. You need to embrace the daily grind and to find pleasure in it. Real progress takes time. It is never a smooth ride. Instead, it's a wobbly path that involves detours, obstacles, and low points along the way to the top.

How you handle those lows determines how long you stay in them. Since failure is a learning opportunity, the champion minded see progress even when they feel they may be regressing. Kevin Anderson, a tennis player from South Africa who reached the top 10 in the world rankings late in his career had this to say about progress, "You need to trust the process and focus on each day. There may be tougher days where you don't feel like you made steps forwards, and that's ok, but there will be other days where you will."

Athletes: there will be times when you are working hard but you don't seem to be moving forward. Know that progress takes time.

Be committed to doing your best each day. Keep working and trusting the process!

Remember that getting better involves consistently putting in the effort while staying patient for the reward. Never rush the process. Trust it!

\* \* \*

*Champion minded athletes*
*know that progress takes time.*
*They invest in the long term journey.*

# Try Again.
# Fail Again.
# Fail Better.

*Champion minded athletes*
*are willing to risk failure in order to succeed.*

T o achieve success, the willingness to take risks and fail is tremendously important. Every aspect of life involves taking risks and failing. Too often people are afraid to fail, afraid to look bad, afraid to be regarded as inadequate, and so, if they do not immediately achieve successful results, they quit trying. Before she went on to pen the best-selling fantasy series in history, twelve publishing houses rejected J.K. Rowling; British novelist, screenwriter, and film producer best known as the author of the Harry Potter series.

The *Kansas City Star* newspaper fired Walt Disney because his editor felt he "lacked imagination and had no good ideas." He went on to acquire Laugh-O-Gram, an animation studio, which then fell into bankruptcy. After these failures, he and his brother moved to California and began the Disney Brothers' Studio, eventually creating Mickey Mouse and Disneyland and winning 22 Academy Awards.

Michael Jordan, arguably the greatest basketball player of all time, was cut from his high school basketball team. Jordan said,

*I have missed over 9,000 shots in my career. I have lost almost 300 games. On 26 occasions I have been entrusted to take the game winning shot and I have missed. I have failed over and over again in my life. And that is why I succeed.*

Athletes - how you respond to failures will either propel you onward, or it will hold you back.

Champion minded athletes respond to failure by learning from losses and trying again. Champion minded athletes persist. When you give yourself permission to fail, you give yourself the opportunity to excel and to innovate. Failure means you are trying new things, learning new things, and pushing yourself beyond past limits.

\* \* \*

*"Ever tried. Ever failed. No matter. Try again. Fail again. Fail better."*

- Samuel Beckett

# Talent is Overrated

*Champion minded athletes work tirelessly and with a good attitude.*

Elite athletes don't just show up and dominate the competition. It takes years of dedication and failing to master a skill. Along the way, there are difficult decisions to make and many challenges to overcome. When it comes to describing a highly skilled athlete, I've never been a huge fan of using the word *talented*. It's a buzz word that gets thrown around too often, and it undervalues the work athletes have put in to get to where there are.

Certainly Roger Federer, Olympic gymnast Simone Biles, and Neymar, Jr. were born with a degree of natural ability, but to attribute their success merely to being talented is to underestimate the countless hours of hard work these athletes have performed upon their journey to the elite levels of their sport. The incredible performers you see on the world stage today shine after many years of blood, sweat and tears.

As the saying goes, "Champions are made when no one is watching." These world-class athletes did not become champions when they held up the first trophy. They became champions during the hours spent relentlessly training, working, and struggling to be in a position to hoist the trophy high.

Athletes - if we are going to talk about talent, then let your habits, attitude, work ethic, coach-ability, resilience, and your hunger to succeed be your greatest attributes. Champion minded athletes work tirelessly and with a good attitude to master skills. Remember that hard work beats talent when talent doesn't work hard.

\* \* \*

*Let your best talent be your work-ethic.*

# There Are No Shortcuts To Success

*Champion minded athletes don't cut corners.*

W hen I observe a warm up, I always look to see if any athletes are cutting corners or stopping just short of the lines. It may seem trivial, but it matters more than you might think. This small detail speaks volumes about the athlete's personal standards, mindset, and level of commitment. The real issue isn't cutting the corner or stopping short of the line. It's what it reveals about your character. The temptation to choose the easiest, quickest, or cheapest way only increases the gap between you and greatness.

Winning is a matter of developing the slight edge. Champion minded athletes put in extra work. Just as it takes time to develop the winning edge, the consequences of cutting corners will gradually set you further and further back.

When training as a young athlete, I was obsessive about doing a little more than my set distance or time. When my training partner called it quits early, it would drive me nuts, because the training time was cut short. One of my mantras, *"Champions do extra,"* kept me from quitting early. It urged me on to put in the extra effort. I was so obsessed with effort, that if I was asked to do a 10 mile run, I would do 10.1 miles just to make sure I'd gone beyond the day's goal. I never understood people who did less.

Tom Graham, an Olympic and world class rowing coach said, "There are no training shortcuts in rowing because races are won by fractions of a second." This is so true! Elite sport is all about little details - inches and milliseconds. Champion minded athletes don't cut corners or stop short of the lines. They choose to put in the extra effort. They are disciplined even when no one is looking.

The champion minded athlete understands there are no shortcuts to success. No athlete who has made it to the top in his or her respective sport ever took the easier/quicker/cheaper way. Although plans vary, one thing all elite plans have in common is this - there are no shortcuts!

* * *

*Champion minded athletes don't cut corners or stop short of the lines. They choose to put in the extra effort. They are disciplined even when no one is looking.*

# Bits & Pieces

*Champion minded athletes
understand the return on small investments.*

I can't emphasize enough the importance of doing what I call the little "bits and pieces." I'm referring to putting in some extra training or stretches when you have some time during the day.

Champion minded athletes capitalize on even the smallest amounts of time they can invest in training. Just a few minutes spent on doing some extra core strengthening exercises or foam rolling, for example, can make a huge difference.

Average athletes don't recognize the value in small bits and pieces of effort. Over an extended period, what might not seem like much at the time, adds up to great rewards and achievement.

Athletes: make the most of your time during and outside of practice and training. Doing the little extras add up to making the big differences in the end.

\* \* \*

*Doing the little extras add up to making the big
differences in the end.*

# You Make Your Own Luck

*Champion minded athletes
create their own luck.*

L uck is a combination of preparation, attitude, and opportunity. The better prepared you are, and the more positive your attitude is, the better your chance for success. When you start to believe less in the ambiguous quality of luck and more in the controllable quality of luck, the luckier you become!

I've found that people who are quick to define themselves as unlucky, are pessimistic thinkers. These types of people focus their energy on what is not going their way and on what could go wrong. Their fatalistic and defeatist outlooks become self-fulfilling prophecies. In other words, they attract it towards themselves. You will also find players under pressure who can sometimes react by blaming events on their "bad luck." They adopt the victim label. They call themselves "unlucky," and they refer to their opponents as "lucky."

Individuals who seem to be lucky share traits of optimism, meticulous preparation, and self-confidence. Their hopeful and positive outlooks become self-fulfilling prophecies.

Champion minded athletes create their own luck by choosing to have a positive attitude, being willing prepare to be successful, and believing in themselves. Hard work leads to good fortune.

So, if someone calls you "lucky," thank them for the compliment. It means you are an optimist and opportunist!

\* \* \*

M

*It's no coincidence that the harder you work,
the luckier you get.*

# Keep a Training Journal

*A training journal helps you stay on track.*

Since age 11, I've kept a training journal. Writing in it each day became a habit I've continued to this day. It gives me a great sense of pride and accomplishment to write down the training I've done each day. I write down what I did well that day and for what I am most grateful. Journaling serves as time for self-reflection and a mini-celebration of small victories. It makes me feel good about myself and it's proven to be a beneficial part of my daily routine.

Keeping a training journal accelerates and deepens the learning process. It is a great tool to track your progress and to identify performance trends and patterns that might otherwise go undetected. I also use it as a reference. When I'm preparing for an event in which I have competed in the past, I like to go back and read what I was doing to get ready at that time and to see what worked or didn't work.

Keeping a training journal helps you track your health and wellness. It assists with keeping track of any nutritional or supplement changes you may have made. Keeping a journal helps you stay in tune with your goals. Creating a record of your hard work and accomplishments builds confidence. Writing down and reviewing your days and weeks of effort helps you feel prepared and ready to compete. It also helps you stay accountable and motivated. Part of tracking progress is being aware of how you are feeling and what you are thinking.

## Benefits of keeping a training journal:

- Helps you monitor your health and wellness
- Tracks your progress
- Keeps a history of your training schedule
- Great way to stay focused on short-term goals and stay motivated for long-term goals
- Builds confidence and pride in the work you've done and effort you've given

\* \* \*

*A journal serves as a great source of motivation and keeps you accountable.*

# The Best are Big on the Small Details

*The champion minded check every box.*

In any given sport, there is no more than a 1% or 2% difference in the skill levels of the top players in the world. Go to a tennis or a golf tournament and watch all of the players practice on the courts or the driving range. If you don't know who the players are, you probably wouldn't be able to tell the difference between the top 10 and the top 100 - they all have world-class skills!

*So what's the difference?*

## There are two key components:

1. Mindset under pressure/control of emotions while competing

2. Superior preparation/attention to detail

Recently I was in Irving, Texas at the Byron Nelson PGA consulting and working with a professional golfer. Among the best golfers, there was former world number one, Jason Day. What stood out about "J-Day" was his attention to detail and his professionalism in absolutely everything he did. Each morning, he ate the same healthy breakfast. After each round of practice, he had his protein shake in hand in the locker room and then he went straight off to the gym to stretch and to perform his regeneration routine. During the entire week, I probably only saw five other guys stretch! Jason was meticulous in everything.

It's easy to see that Jason lives like a professional. He is an example of someone who has maximized his potential by taking care of the small things. Some might say, "So, big deal, he stretches and has a recovery shake!"  But, it's in these little things, done consistently everyday where success happens.

When I asked Greg Gaultier, the world number 1 player in Squash (at time of print), what he felt was the key to success, he said, "Loving what you do and being good with the small details. It's not only about how I spend my time on the court, but off it to."

Athletes: practicing and working on your game represents only 20% of your week. Success occurs during the other 80% of the time. Become world-class in the 80% of your time spent away from the court, field, or course. Be *Champion Minded*.

\* \* \*

*It's in the small things, done consistently everyday, where success happens.*

*Success is a result of consistently doing the small things with effort over an extended period of time.*

*Success = Time + Consistent Effort*

# Master the Fundamentals

*Champion minded athletes
are great at the fundamentals.*

C hampion minded athletes diligently and meticulously practice fundamentals. In his book, "The Talent Code," Daniel Coyle describes this as "mastering the mundane," doing the boring work with monomaniacal focus and purpose. It's impossible to reach world-class levels without having world-class fundamentals.

Michael Jordan credits his accomplishments to the coaches who taught him to master the fundamentals. Jordan said,

> *I had to learn the fundamentals of basketball, because you can have all the physical ability in the world, but you still need to know the fundamentals. I discovered early on that the player who learned the fundamentals of basketball was going to have a much better chance of succeeding and rising through the levels of competition than the player who was content to do things his own way. A player should be interested in learning why things are done a certain way. The reasons behind the teaching often go a long way to helping develop the skill.*

Athletes: the quality of your habits under pressure reflect your grasp of the fundamentals. It is absolutely essential to learn, develop, and appreciate the fundamentals. They should be practiced in every session. Of fundamentals, world-renowned sports performance coach, Mark Verstegen says, "success is in doing the simple things savagely well." A distinguishing factor between the good and the great is their mastery of the fundamentals.

Fundamentals keep things simple. The New Zealand All Blacks rugby program provides a great example. The All Blacks do nothing revolutionary. They stick to the basics and the fundamentals and do them better than anyone else.

\* \* \*

*"I discovered early on that the player who learned the fundamentals was going to have a much better chance of succeeding."*

- Michael Jordan

*Everyone wants to be great until it's time to do what greatness requires.*

# Repetition, Repetition, Repetition

*Champion minded athletes
are committed to repetition.*

Repetition is key to mastering skill. The athlete's relationship with repetition is a major factor separating the good from the great. Mastery involves comprehensive knowledge and proficiency of a skill. Athletes: mastery is not attained from working until you get it right once, mastery is attained by continued repetition until you can't get it wrong. Champion minded athletes are committed to repetition to achieve mastery of a skill.

Recently on a training run, I was listening to a podcast featuring master chef and restaurateur, Thomas Keller. When asked what it takes to be a successful chef, he answered, "A great chef needs to be in love with repetition, which I am. It's about doing the same thing every day at a consistent and high level." He explained further, suggesting producing one great meal does not make a great chef or restaurant, but rather, consistently producing great meals is what takes one to the top in the world of cuisine.

Athletes: purposeful repetition means committing a great level of focus and effort into every swing, pitch, kick, row, tackle, serve, and shot you perform in each practice. Going through the motions does not lead to greatness. Purposeful repetition leads to greatness. Toni Nadal, uncle and coach of grand slam champion and world number one Rafael Nadal, has said that there were many other tennis players with more talent than Rafael. Rafael's commitment to repetition with fierce intensity and extreme focus helped him achieve success at the highest level of tennis competition.

Tom Brady is regarded as one of the greatest NFL quarterbacks of all time. When asked what he thought was the key to his development from an average high school and college player to a multiple Super Bowl winning quarterback, he responded, "I practiced harder than anyone I knew. I was also great at handling repetition and spending countless hours perfecting my throwing technique." Repetition alone does not produce elite athletes. Champion minded athletes approach repetition with a deep understanding and purposeful commitment.

\* \* \*

*"A baseball swing is a very finely tuned instrument.*
*It is repetition, and more repetition,*
*and then a little more after that."*

\- Reggie Jackson

*Your effort level is a direct reflection of your interest level. You don't need to tell everyone how invested you are, your actions will do that.*

# Master the Mundane

## *Champion minded athletes embrace purposeful repetition.*

I first encountered the term "mastering the mundane" in Daniel Coyle's book, *The Talent Code.* In his book, Coyle explores where talent comes from and how it is developed. Why are so many great soccer players from Brazil? How does a poor financed tennis club in Moscow produce more top 20 women's players than anywhere else in the world? Why does the Boishoi Ballet School produce the world's best dancers?

Coyle identifies a commitment to mastering fundamentals as a key trait among talent hotbeds. Though this seems mundane, it is accurate. These athletes are not necessarily the most naturally talented, but they develop skill by dedicating themselves to mastering the fundamentals. Performing a skill once or twice does not indicate mastery. Performing a skill repeatedly and consistently signifies mastery. To reach a level of unconscious competence, to perform a skill consistently without having to concentrate to achieve it, to just do it without having to think about it, is to master the mundane. This takes a long time. Champion minded athletes commit the time to master the mundane. It's a long-term commitment to excellence.

To master the mundane and to reach unconscious competence, practice must be mindful, not mindless. Mindful practice is practice with a purpose. Mindless practice simply passes the time. The commitment to staying mindful during practice trains the skill to stay mentally tough during competition.

Reaching the top in any field requires a commitment to mastering the fundamentals and to keeping focused throughout the process. Every athlete loves to play. It is the champion minded athlete who masters the mundane.

\* \* \*

*The mastering of a skill involves a more mindful and deeper relationship with repetition.*

*You can tell the average athletes from the champion minded ones when you demand excellence from them. The average hate it, the champion minded love it!*

# Otra Vez

### *The champion minded keep trying.*

I recently watched a video of a great coach working with a group of young Spanish athletes. He kept repeating, "Otra vez, otra vez!" His students responded by trying - again and again. He explained the drill clearly and concisely in the beginning, and then simply urged them to try again and again.

Listening to an interview on the Tim Ferris podcast, I was reminded of this video. Tim was interviewing American snowboarder and Olympic gold medalist, Shaun White. When asked about his secret to success, Shaun explained that there was no secret. He just kept trying and trying - again and again.

When the subject changed to his training habits and to how he learned a new move, Shaun replied that he would spend hours and hours getting that one move right until he could no longer get it wrong. This is an incredible example of a growth mindset and a champion mindset! Undeterred by failure, he kept at it - again and again. He continued on to say that the amazing trick moves seen on TV were the combined result of his many failures, his refusal to quit and his resolve to keep trying again and again. He explained, "This is what most people don't see. They just see the amazing stuff you do and think you're just a natural. This couldn't be further from the truth."

Athletes frequently give up too soon. They fail a few times and they abandon the attempt to try again. Sometimes progress happens quickly. Most often, however, progress is slow.  Keep trying.  You'll get it.  You can do it.  *Otra vez, otra vez!*

\* \* \*

*The champion minded understand that success takes time, persistence, and an incredible amount of failing.*

# The Separation is in the Preparation

*Everyday the champion minded prepare to win.*

The higher you rise in the ranks of your chosen sport, the tougher the competition becomes. Like the proverb states, "it gets tougher at the top." The field narrows - everyone has sound fundamentals, everyone is physically fit, everyone is paying attention to their nutrition and hydration. Most are paying attention to the small details. So what's the distinguishing factor? We return to the question of what separates the good from the great.

It's your daily work ethic, habits, and standards that are going to separate you from the rest of the field. Natural talent is great, but attitude and work ethic determine how far you go. You are in control of your preparation. Take charge of the day and be accountable. Schedule your bedtime and wake time. Pack your bag the night before your competition. Maintain your equipment. Prepare your meals/snacks ahead of time. Hydrate. Eat a healthy breakfast. Give 100% effort in practice and competition. Do what is right even when no one is watching. Do more without being asked. Discipline yourself so someone else doesn't have to.

Kevin Anderson, who has reached the top 10 in the world, is a player I've worked with since 2014. He said this about the importance of preparing well, "It's about putting in the hours and being smart about your preparation. Especially now, I put an extra emphasis on taking care of my body. You need to be structured and professional off the court too when it comes to things like your nutrition, hydration intake, your daytime naps, etc."

Football coach Vince Lombardi phrased it well, "The will to win is not nearly so important as the will to prepare to win." Most people have the will to win. Most people enjoy winning and all that comes with it. The people willing to put in the "hard work over time" required to prepare to win are far more rare. Great performers have that rare will to prepare. What makes this challenging is that it's not a one-time thing. You can't prepare to win once and then just let success flow. Great performers have the will to prepare over and over again. The champion minded set themselves up for success by always being well prepared.

* * *

*"The will to win is not nearly so important as the will to prepare to win."*

- Vince Lombardi

# 10 Daily Habits of A Champion

## *Champion minded athletes have world class habits.*

Athletes: the choices you make everyday contribute to your long-term success. To produce consistent performance and better results, champion minded athletes have routines in place. They operate best when they have structure to their days and priorities in place.

## Champion minded athletes:

1. **have a set wake time and are early risers:** Sleep is vital to performance. Champion minded athletes aim to get 7-9 hours each night.

2. **have a morning motivational reading:** Champion minded athletes prepare themselves mentally by scheduling time at the start of the day for motivational or spiritual reading, which facilitates calm, strength, and encouragement.

3. **have a large and healthy breakfast:** By providing energy and alertness, a healthy breakfast prepares the body and the mind for the day.

4. **pre-plan meals:** Nutrition is key to performance. To stay on track throughout the day, champions eat like champions and prepare healthy choices in advance.

5. **pack their bag the night before:** Preparing gear and equipment the night before gives peace of mind, which enhances sleep quality and reduces morning stress.

6. **schedule regeneration time at home:** Champion minded athletes follow regularly scheduled recovery routines (foam rolling, stretching, etc.).

7. **stay hydrated throughout the day:** Sipping water throughout the day keeps your body hydrated - this is of utmost importance! Hydration aids recovery, energy levels, and mental focus. Sipping regularly is better than drinking large amounts sporadically.

8. **take daily naps:** Champion minded athletes believe in the power of daytime naps. Naps help recovery. Naps help relax and refresh the athlete for the training session, helping prepare them to maximize practice, especially if there are multiple sessions each day (morning and afternoon).

9. **have good communication skills:** Champion minded athletes plan ahead. They coordinate with coaches, trainers, parents, and teachers about practice times, training sessions, competition calendar, school homework and testing schedule, transportation, equipment maintenance, nutrition, and hydration.

10. **have winning self-talk:** Champion minded athletes understand that their inner thoughts and self-talk are the key to a more successful and a happier life.

# Competitive Training

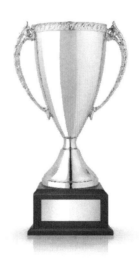

# Mental Toughness:
# Foundational & Competitive

*Mental toughness in sports starts with your daily discipline in life.*

The more I work with high level sports performers the more evident the following becomes: competitive mental toughness on the field, on the court, or on the course, originates from your foundational mental toughness - the discipline you have in your daily habits and lifestyle.

When an athlete asks me to help them with their mental game, my first action is to observe the discipline and the structure of their foundation - their lifestyle habits. Improving the athlete's daily habits, are the first steps toward improving the player. Once the athlete has improved their lifestyle habits and strengthen foundational mental toughness, we can focus on competitive mental toughness.

Competitive mental toughness is not just about pushing through tough workouts, fighting hard and never giving up. It's about building the right habits and staying disciplined on a day to day basis. In order to develop true mental toughness, you need structure to your day.

The people athletes choose to surround themselves with, especially their significant others, play a critical role in an athlete's performance. For an athlete to develop the right mindset and purpose, coaches, teammates, family, and supporters all need to be on the same page.

I can easily see the level of discipline in someone's lifestyle. A glance at the following reveals much about a person's character. Is their living space a mess? If so, I already know that other things in their lifestyle may also be disorganized and messy. Are they always running late for appointments or practices? Though this might seem minor, it displays a lack of planning and self-discipline that contributes to foundational mental toughness.

Digging deep in competition, continuing to fight and to stay focused when fatigue and stress set in, and staying positive when difficulty arises, are all key components of competitive mental toughness. Competitive mental toughness skills originate from foundational mental toughness skills, which include staying disciplined in your day-to-day routines and consistently managing good habits while maintaining a positive attitude. When you are able to achieve this over a longer period of time, that's when you'll experience the greater rewards.

* * *

*Competitive mental toughness originates from foundational mental toughness.*

*Building mental muscle is like building physical muscle. It requires a concerted effort and takes time. The more you do of it, the better you become at it.*

# Monkeys & Gorillas

*Develop the right mindset in practice
in order to compete successfully.*

In the past, I've consulted with athletes who think it's acceptable to be negative during practice, believing that when it's time to compete, they'll be more positive. They believe that the negativity, poor body language, and poor energy they display in practice isn't relevant to their competitive performance. They could not be more wrong!

They let their monkeys (their negative emotions and reactions) loose during practice time, lacking the self-control or the focus to tame them.

During competition, you don't rise to your expectations, you fall back on the quality of your habits. What you do in practice is crucial. If you behave with negativity, mumbling, and poor body language during practice, then these detrimental tendencies will come visit you like a big fat ugly gorilla during competition.

Just like your game skills, your mindset skills need to be trained and developed. If you don't display positive energy on the practice court or field, thinking you're going to be positive and portray great energy when you compete is just wishful thinking.

I always like to remind my athletes, "If you're not confronting your monkeys in practice, then expect a visit from the big fat ugly gorillas during competition."

\* \* \*

M

*You won't get it right under pressure during competition if you haven't practiced getting it right under pressure in practice.*

*You can't expect above average results with a below average mindset.*

# What If?

*Have a plan for every possible scenario that could go wrong.*

I like to play a game with my athletes called *"what if?"* If refers to the possibility of something going wrong in a match or a race and questions how they would respond to it.

The best and most successful athletes in the world are the most prepared to compete. In the words of former USA Track star and Olympic gold medalist, Michael Johnson, "Preparation is everything."

The best of the best are all prepared for the unexpected. They have covered every possible scenario that could go wrong, and have a plan in place. A great example of this comes from Michael Phelps, the most decorated swimmer in Olympic history, when he was competing in the 2008 Olympics in Beijing. During the race, his goggles began to fill with water, forcing him to race almost blind for the remaining 175 meters of the race. Phelps said that he felt relaxed and didn't panic since, many times in practice, he had already prepared for something like this happening. Tennis champion Roger Federer says, "It's all in the details," referring to the little things that could go wrong and being mentally prepared for them. These champion minded athletes have a ready response to adversity.

A few years back, I had a chat over dinner with the motorsport principal of a touring car racing team. He explained that an enormous amount of time was devoted to putting strategies in place to handle any possible scenario that could arise on the track during a race. They covered every problem and developed solutions for what could go wrong: electronic failures, a headset malfunctioning, tire blowouts, weather changes, driver penalties, the list goes on and on. If you can think of a potential problem, they have a solution. This is a great example of how the best are the best-prepared to succeed in high pressure and intensely competitive environments.

Champion minded athletes visualize themselves performing well and responding to possible obstacles with courage and calmness. By facing the reality of adversity, they rehearse being tested, train pushing their limits, and are never caught unaware or surprised by an unforeseen circumstance. With a positive attitude, champion minded athletes hope for the best, are not discouraged by the worst, and are prepared for everything in between.

* * *

*Adversity on the course is inevitable. Don't train to avoid it, plan for it, train for it and prepare for it.*

*Nothing will slow down your progress like a negative mindset.*
*Like a flat tire, it will get you nowhere until you change it.*

# Adopt The "1 More" Mentality

*Champion minded athletes
do the extra for themselves.*

From a young age, if I was asked to do a certain number of repetitions, or run for a certain amount of time, I would perform an extra rep or add on a few seconds. For example; if I was asked to do 10 push-ups, I'd do 11. If I was asked to run for 20 minutes, I'd run for 21.

I wasn't doing it to please my coach or my supporters. I wanted to do that extra rep for me. I knew that if I could just give extra effort in everything I did, then over time I'd improve and I'd get better than my opponents. Believe it or not, it wasn't as difficult as you might imagine.

At a young age, I already had that "gain the slight edge" mentality in operation. I put in the little extras everyday, and then watched those efforts accumulate into bigger results.

Be champion minded. Do one more rep - for you!

\* \* \*

*No coach or person can make you great if you're not
willing to put in the hard work.*

# Champion Work Ethic

*Champion minded athletes
have a world-class work ethic.*

Hard work leads to excellence in sport. The best athletes in their sports work hard without having to always be pushed. They lead, they motivate, and they hold themselves accountable.

Pat Kerney worked himself to greatness. After walking-on and playing college football at the University of Virginia, he became the first-round draft pick of the Atlanta Falcons in 1999. Then, while with the Seattle Seahawks in 2007, Pat was voted as a Pro bowl starter. During his time as head coach of the Falcons, Jim L. Mora said of Kerney:

> *The great ones hold themselves to a higher standard. What's made them great is that they consistently give tremendous all-out effort. They hold themselves accountable on every play. Some players might ease up on a few plays, but the great ones, they never take a day off. In Pat's case, he refuses to relent. He can go and go and go and go. I think most of the great ones have that relentlessness.*

Kobe Bryant also worked himself to greatness. In the summer of 2012, a professional trainer named Rob was hired to train the USA basketball team which would be competing in the London Olympics. In his first meeting with Kobe, Rob discussed his areas of specialization and where Kobe would like to be physically at the end of the summer. Rob then gave Kobe his number and told him to contact him if he wanted to put in some additional conditioning work. Two days later, Kobe called Rob at 4:15am.

"Hey, uhh Rob, I hope I'm not disturbing anything right?"

"Uhh no, what's up Kobe?"

"Just wondering if you could just help me out with some conditioning work, that's all."

"Yeah sure, I'll see you in the facility in a bit."

20 minutes later, Rob arrived at the training facility. There, he saw Kobe, alone and drenched in so much sweat it looked like he'd just come from a pool. It was not even 5:00am yet! The two of them worked on conditioning for about 75 minutes, then did 45 minutes of weight training. At 7am, Rob went back to his hotel to get some rest before the day's practice. Meanwhile, Kobe went back to the gym to practice his shooting. Rob was expected back at 11am. He slept a couple of hours, got a quick breakfast, and then headed back to the gym exhausted and sleep deprived. When he arrived, he saw all of the members of Team USA there. LeBron was talking to Carmelo. Coach Krzyzewski was explaining something to Kevin Durant, and on the right side of the facility, all by himself, Kobe was shooting jumpers.

Rob went up to Kobe and said, "Good work this morning."

"Huh?"

"Like, the conditioning. Good work."

"Oh. Yeah, thanks Rob. I really appreciate it."

"So when did you finish?"

"Finish what?"

"Getting your shots up. What time did you leave the facility?"

"Oh just now. I wanted 800 makes...so yeah, just now."

Rob's jaw dropped. Kobe was drenched in sweat before 5:00am, worked with Rob on strength and conditioning for 2 hours, then made 800 shots between the hours of 7:00am and 11:00am. And this all took place before practice!

A great example of a champion minded work ethic and mentality.

* * *

*Even still at 34 years of age and with 5 NBA championships, Kobe was still waking up before 4am and working out for a few hours before team practice even began!*

*"There are many things I want, and the only way I will get them is to keep my head down, listen to the right people, and work hard."*

- Mia Hamm

# 15-90

## *Small efforts add up to great achievements.*

I first learned about the 15-90 theory after watching a video on YouTube featuring American gymnast and Olympic medalist, Peter Vidmar. Now retired, Vidmar won gold medals in the men's all-around team competition and the pommel horse competition, as well as a silver medal in the men's all-around individual gymnastics competition at the 1984 Summer Olympic Games in Los Angeles.

Peter did the extra work. Like all champion minded athletes, Peter was determined to be great. He realized that by doing what his coaches asked, he could be good. But, in order to be great, he needed to do more. Driven to succeed, Peter believed that if he spent at least 15 minutes in extra training per day, he could gain a slight edge. He would be that much closer to achieving his goals. He realized that doing just 15 minutes extra each day would add up to 90 hours per year! After winning the gold medal, Peter credited the habit of putting in 15 extra minutes of effort per day as the differentiator between him and his competitors.

Champion minded athletes are willing to do the extra work. Golfer Jason Day, soccer star Ronaldo, Olympic gymnast Madison Kocian, or the rugby great Dan Carter, are all great examples of individuals who are well known to put in the extra efforts when the rest had called it a day. After practices, they worked tirelessly on improving their skills.

If you want to be great, you have to be willing to put in the extra work. In the end, it's the extra work which makes the difference.

\* \* \*

*"When you improve a little each day, eventually big things occur... Not tomorrow, not the next day, but eventually a big gain is made."*

\- John Wooden

# Luck

*Champion minded athletes
create their own luck.*

When I hear people bemoan their misfortune and say that a certain team or an individual is "so lucky," I have to chuckle. A team or an individual is lucky because they are prepared, because they believe in their abilities and skills, because they stay positive, because they take risks, and because aren't afraid to fail.

Luck is a self-fulfilling prophesy. If you are always complaining that you never win anything, you won't win. If you tell yourself that you always choke, you're going to choke. If you tell yourself you can't beat a certain opponent, you won't beat them.

Luck favors the prepared, the optimists, and the hard workers. Preparation and luck are inseparable concepts because luck rarely finds the person who is unprepared for the opportunity that might come their way. In the words of legendary Coach John Wooden, "When the opportunity arises, it is too late to prepare."

I've also discovered that athletes who thrive in sports, where luck plays a modest role, are excellent problem solvers, are able to separate effort from result, and they bounce back quickly when the cards don't fall in their favor.

While the unlucky are busy complaining about their misfortunes, the champion minded are working to create their own good luck. You work yourself lucky. It's as simple as that!

\* \* \*

*"It's a funny thing.*
*The more I practice, the luckier I get."*

- Arnold Palmer

# Drive & Determination

*The more you are willing to risk and fail,
the closer you are to greatness.*

Growing up, I had a vision and a goal to represent my country at the world championships in Duathlon (running and cycling). Sometimes that goal would keep me awake at night. Although I was never the best in my age group - far from it - I felt like I was getting better every year. I was getting closer to the kids that had always been better than I was and closing that gap motivated me to work even harder. Early on, I realized I was not as talented as the others, but I was more driven and determined. Rather than the best athlete award, I always wanted to win the "most improved athlete" award at my club. I was fixated on bettering myself. Being the "best player" meant I was being compared to others, but being the most improved meant I was competing with myself.

After missing selections and failing many times, I never quit. It was through those failures that I developed the toughness to endure obstacles and embrace struggles. Finally, at age 18, I made my first national team to compete in the world championships. That same year, I also won a junior national title, and captained the national team. Without even knowing it, I had been building grit and leadership skills.

I made it a point to always work a little harder than my training partners. My relentless work ethic raised my adrenaline and became my biggest motivation If we were going for a 3 hour training ride, I'd do an extra 15 or 20 minutes. In the gym, after everyone had gone, I'd do a few extra core or strength exercises. I believed that a little extra effort would add up and bring me closer to my vision and goal. I went on to compete in 5 world championships, claimed 3 national titles, and signed a pro contract with a professional team in Europe.

Winning margins at the Olympics can be minuscule. The athletes who win by an inch, a hundredth of a second, or one point, didn't get to the podium by chance. They all had the drive and determination to do a little extra. A champion minded athlete understands that talent is not everything. What counts most is drive and determination to succeed. Let your opponents motivate you to work harder. I'm grateful that I wasn't the most talented young athlete or a prodigy. Learning to work hard, to have self-discipline, to believe in myself, to be driven and determined - these traits have helped me in sport and in life. The same can apply to you as well. The question is: How bad do you want it?

* * *

*Hard work beats talent when talent doesn't work hard.*

# The Only Thing Constant in Life is Change

*Getting to the top is one thing;*
*staying at the top it quite another.*

When a player makes a change in their game, performance usually gets worse before it gets better. Thus, players are often resistant to change. They reach a certain level of success with a skill and they don't want to make the necessary changes because of the initial lack of success. This is short-sighted. Athletes: avoid becoming satisfied or complacent with your skill set due to current successes. It's so important to continue to make changes in areas of technique, tactics, and training, etc.. What you've done to reach a certain level of success in your sport does not mean you've done enough to keep you at that level. It's certainly not enough to get you to the next level. Your opponents will eventually figure out your strengths and weaknesses, and they'll go to work on them.

Champion minded athletes constantly evolve. They are not content to do only what they've always done. Athletes who resist change - who are not willing to suffer through the growing pains of change - are the athletes who are ultimately left behind. Sometimes circumstances like an injury or illness, force an athlete to make a change. Sometimes it takes disappointing results to bring about a "crisis management" change. The champion minded are always setting themselves up for success. They change before they have to.

Roger Federer dominated tennis for more than a decade. Even after achieving record-breaking success, he realized he needed to make changes to continue to compete at the highest level. Federer added additional coaches and trainers to his team, changed racquets, altered his fitness program, and updated his on-court competitive techniques and tactics.

Three-time Olympic beach volleyball gold medalist, Misty May Treanor, said, "I recognized that skill and talent got us to the top, but it wouldn't keep us there. So, we had to plan accordingly. We had to be willing to try new things to keep winning. You have to be open to new approaches."

What got you to a certain level won't necessarily get you to the next. The champion minded know that to achieve their fullest potential, they must be willing to step away from their comfort zone and embrace change.

* * *

*Champion minded athletes embrace change and aim to continually improve and evolve.*

# Present Yourself as A Champion

*Champions look like champions.*

onfidence is the best accessory to any outfit. Champions have a particular swagger, a certain way they carry themselves that sets them apart and makes them easily recognizable. Roger Federer, Alison Felix, Cristiano Ronaldo, Usian Bolt, and Tom Brady come to mind. Yes, it's easier to be fashionably put together when backed by million dollar contracts and endorsement deals, but it doesn't take millions to look professional and to carry yourself like a champion. When you look like a million bucks, you feel like a million bucks, but it doesn't take a million bucks!

Throughout his golf career, Tiger Woods famously wore red shirts on Sundays (final rounds of tournaments). In the "Dear Tiger" section of his website, in which he responds to fans' questions, Woods explained his wardrobe selection as such, "I wear red on Sundays because my mom thinks that that's my power color." Woods began wearing red in final rounds even before turning professional.

Andre Agassi brought a new sense of fashion and attitude to men's professional tennis in the 1980's and 90's. In his iconic TV commercial for Canon in 1990, Agassi coined the phrase, "Image is everything." Similarly, Muhammad Ali said, "I am the greatest. I said that even before I knew I was." Present yourself as a champion even before you are one.

How we dress impacts how we feel and perform. If you play a team sport, then you obviously don't decide what colors you will wear. However, if you play an individual sport, then prepare to have your favorite gear and colors ready to wear in competition. This will help you feel confident and energized. Your appearance is one of your standards.  Make the effort to look your best as part of your preparation to perform at your best. Remember, that a champion minded athlete looks like a winner!

* * *

*How you present yourself significantly affects how others see you and how you see yourself.*

# Control Your Body Language

*Confident athletes display a great aura through their body language.*

I have been in the locker rooms and warm up areas of champion minded athletes such as Roger Federer, Novak Djokovic, and many other sports stars. I can honestly tell you that they are feeling the pressure - the butterflies in the stomach, the gripping tightness.... But, being champion minded, their body language does not necessarily reflect how they feel inside. While they may feel anxious and nervous on the inside, outwardly they communicate confidence and readiness.

Your opponent cannot read your mind. But, they can observe your body language, and it speaks volumes. Regularly practice controlling your body language. Just as negative body language communicates fear, defeat, lack of will, frustration, and lack of interest; positive body language powerfully communicates confidence, belief, grit, and a fighting spirit. Positive posture may intimidate your opponent, unnerve them, or increase their fear and self-doubt. Negative posture emboldens your opponent, making them feel more secure in their quest for victory.

Positive or negative, your body language exposes your thoughts and feelings. It communicates a clear message to others - your opponent, team members, coaches, parents, and spectators.

Champion minded athletes understand the importance of controlling their body language and how it affects their performance and results.

* * *

*Your opponent can't read your mind,*
*but they can read your body language.*

*Your opponent feeds off of your poor body language & negativity - they are inspired & energized by it.*

*Protect it!*

# Why Warm-Ups Matter

*Preparing for peak performance.*

Anyone who is familiar with the McCaw Method knows that I'm a stickler for purposeful, high-quality warm-ups. *It all matters - details, details, details!*

Before every practice and competition there should be a warm-up. Athletes: it's of great importance to know *how* and *why* to warm up properly. Developing a warm-up routine that is specific to your needs and to the demands of your sport is imperative. Whether or not your coach is present, you need to be committed and disciplined enough to perform your own warm-up. Legendary Coach John Wooden took notes about his players while they were warming-up. Wooden viewed every detail, including the warm up, as an opportunity to gain a slight edge.

I love attending live sporting events. I particularly enjoy arriving early enough to watch the athletes warm up. I've observed some of the very best in the world, and they leave absolutely nothing to chance.

## 5 Reasons Why Warm-Ups Matter:

1. Better Performance - You need to be physically and mentally ready right from the start.

2. Injury Prevention - Once warmed up, your body has a greater range of motion and more flexibility. Rehearsing movement patterns gets blood pumping which loosens muscles and lubricates joints. Breathing becomes faster and deeper, allowing

the breathing in of more oxygen and the breathing out of more carbon dioxide. A rise in heart rate delivers more oxygen and glucose to the muscles for energy production. A rise in body temperature means you will start sweating.

3. Improved Coordination - As your body warms up, there are more efficient signal transfers along motor nerves; meaning muscles, ligaments, and tendons work together more smoothly when they are elongated and elastic.

4. Mental Focus - Following a specific routine eliminates distraction and enhances concentration. It gets you locked in and focused.

5. Emotional Control - Your standards, discipline, and your commitment in the preparation leading up to the competition, build your confidence. Following a warm-up routine is the final stage of preparation. It boosts belief and calms nerves.

*Warm-up like a champion!*

# Train with Those Who Push You to Be Better

*Champion minded athletes
seek better practice partners.*

The environment you choose and the people you surround yourself with are two of the most important decisions you will make. People tend to take on the traits of the people with whom they spend the most time. Like-minded people tend to gravitate to each other. This is how fraternities, sororities, clubs, communities, fellowships, guilds, unions, churches, and societies form - groups start with common interests and beliefs. Choose your connections and associations carefully. Choose your practice partners carefully. Champion minded athletes set themselves apart from those with lesser standards. Champion minded athletes seek practice partners who will push them past their comfort zones.

Champion minded athletes choose practice partners who challenge them to be better. By choosing a stronger, more experienced, more disciplined, more accomplished, or more skilled practice partner, you give yourself the opportunity to raise your standards and your training capacity. Athletes learn and develop skills through deliberate practice. When you have the opportunity to train with a great practice partner, give your best effort. From their habits and routines, to their exercises and drills, watch, listen, and absorb all there is to learn. Work hard with an open mind and a positive attitude. When given the opportunity to be the better practice partner, give back with patience, kindness, and humility.

Be proactive and make the effort to reach out to other athletes or their coaches to set up practice. This may include traveling beyond your local area to train. I knew an athlete who lived in Wales, but traveled four times a week to the northern part of England to train with better athletes. By car, the trip totaled four hours! However, he was determined to train with the best, so he could become the best. Champion minded athletes make the extra effort to train with better practice partners.

* * *

*To become the best, you need to train with the best.*

*If you're not competing and practicing your hardest, you're cheating yourself. Win or lose, it doesn't matter. What matters most is the effort you give.*

# Need-To-Do vs Nice-To-Do

*Champion minded athletes*
*continually tweak their routines.*

We are all are creatures of habit. I find it amusing to see the same people at the gym at the same time, doing the same class, machine, or routine, day in and day out. They have settled into a comfortable routine, or what they like to do and feel successful doing. Maybe there were initial results, but these folks eventually plateau and experience frustration due to a lack of continued results. This reminds me of Albert Einstein's definition of insanity, "doing the same thing over and over again and expecting different results."

Champion minded athletes regularly assess their training programs, routines, and habits. They then see if there are any areas that might need changes in order to continually improve and to see results. When you feel comfortable, it's time to assess, to make adjustments, and to get uncomfortable. We enjoy doing activities in which we are successful and tend to avoid activities in which we are not successful. It's simply more fun to do what you are good at doing. Usually, what you need to do is what you are avoiding doing due to a lack of success, which leads to a lack of enjoyment.

Champion minded athletes spend time on what they need to do, not just what they enjoy doing. It's a discipline and awareness that they have and live by. They are willing to do what is needed, not just what is comfortable. Avoiding the *"need-to-do"* drills and exercises will in the long term be a costly mistake. Remember, when you're cruising, your losing!

* * *

*Don't fall in to the trap of spending too much time on the "nice stuff." It's usually the things you don't like to do that are needed most in order to improve.*

# When the Going Gets Tough

*Champion minded athletes
keep going when the going gets tough.*

Athletes: the choices you make everyday ultimately define the person you become. You are either going forwards or you are going backwards. There is no in between. Staying comfortable is definitely less challenging and less demanding than continually pushing yourself beyond your current limits. Staying inside your comfort zone certainly takes less effort, but you get what you give - the greater the effort you give, the greater the reward you earn.

The response to criticism and adversity is a major distinguishing factor between champion minded athletes and the rest. You've probably heard the saying, "When the going gets tough, the tough get going" - it's so true! It's easy to say you want to be the best, but when it's time to get up early, when your coach is demanding more of you, when your trainer is pushing you to do an extra rep, when the playing conditions are not ideal, when you are struggling to perform, or when you have to miss a social event, do your decisions and actions reflect your desire to be the best? You may say you want to be the best, but are you doing what it takes?

When faced with challenges, champion minded athletes persist. They appreciate the unique demands of practice, training, and competing. They invite any opportunity to build resilience and grit. They may not enjoy every aspect, but they maintain the discipline to keep going when they are uncomfortable. They know that pushing their limits leads to improvement and better performance. When faced with adversity, persistence is an attitude. Attitude is your choice. Choose to get uncomfortable and choose to be champion minded.

* * *

*"You're not going to enjoy every minute of the journey, but the success you'll find at the end will make it all worth it."*

- Muhammad Ali

# Prepare Under Pressure

*Champion minded athletes
train in pressure situations to simulate play.*

W<br>e all know that person who is a superstar in practice, but who totally chokes in competition. Teams and individuals can crumble under pressure. A few weeks ago, at a USA basketball youth workshop in Chicago, I was speaking to a coach who told me about one of his players who shoots more than 80% in practice, but less than 37% in competition. Is that a technical skill issue? I don't think so. Mental? You bet! If he can do it in practice, then why can't he do it in a game?

You don't rise to your level when put under pressure. Instead, you revert to the habits you have developed during practice time. In other words, your habits (good or bad) during practice time, reveal themselves when placed under stress or adversity. Learning how to develop those better habits requires a concerted effort during your practices.

In order to simulate competition and to challenge their limits, champion minded athletes push themselves to their limits during training. In an interview featuring women's beach volleyball 3-time Olympic gold medalist, Kerri Walsh Jennings, she said, "It all comes down to handling the pressure moments better. At the top, the best are so close in skills and game intelligence, however, I believe what separates the best from the rest, is their ability to handle pressure moments better." Walsh also went onto to add that their Brazilian coach often had them practice under pressure situations.

While observing sports training programs around the world, I've noticed relatively little time is spent having to perform under pressure. Then, when the critical moment arrives, the athlete lacks experience in performing under pressure and is more likely to underachieve.

Champion minded athletes don't just practice their reps. They practice performing the reps under pressure. During practice time, they develop good habits and proper thinking patterns. These are tools for success.

* * *

*The champion minded*
*handle the pressure moments better.*

*To perform under pressure, you have to push your limits and perform under pressure in practice.*

# Live the Best Story of Your Life

*The story you tell yourself becomes your reality.*

A few years ago I was in Tucson, Arizona speaking at a conference. Between my own speaking engagements, I had the opportunity to attend and to listen to my good friend, Bob Litwin speak about the stories we tell ourselves. Bob is an amazing person and the author of *Live the Best Story of Your Life*. Bob's book was all about how your inner beliefs shape your reality and how they eventually become the story of your life.

Inner dialogue often takes on story form. How we tell ourselves these stories, replaying and recreating situations and conversations in our minds, is incredibly important. Champion minded people use positive self-talk in their inner dialogue. Positive self-talk is a product of an optimistic mindset, a hopeful outlook, and grateful attitude. Athletes - is your inner dialogue positive, affirming, and encouraging? Or is it negative, cynical, and defeatist? Positive self-talk is fundamental to success. The stories we tell ourselves in our inner dialogues become either positive or negative fuel.

All too frequently, I've witnessed athletes and individuals hinder their own progress through damaging self-talk. They always seem to revert back to their 'old story'. The truth is, you can talk yourself into or out of almost anything. Defeatist stories in your mind will ensure defeat in reality. You write your own story. Why not write a champion's ending? Unless you create new stories or re-write old stories, you'll continue to relive past endings.

Champion minded athletes maintain the highest standards in their inner dialogue. They are disciplined in practicing positive self-talk. Tell yourself a new story today. The past is in the past. Leave it there, and leave any detrimental, destructive, and harmful self-talk behind. Write your new story today and live it!

\* \* \*

*"The bars you set and reach, both high and low, are connected to the stories you tell yourself."*

-Bob Litwin

# Champions Do More

*Greatness comes from giving extra effort.*

The All Blacks rugby team has a great philosophy and culture. One of their 15 principles states "Champions Do Extra." Being the most successful team in world sport, with a winning record over every rugby team on the planet, the slogan may explain a big part of the reason why. At the start of 2016, I was able to cross off one of my bucket list items. I visited the home of New Zealand rugby, Eden Park. Walking through the corridors and stepping onto the field, I sensed the incredibly powerful history built on the culture and the standards of the All Blacks.

I've worked with athletes of all levels of ability and experience, from those with little natural talent, to those who are very skilled, and from junior players just starting to compete, to gold medal winning Olympians. The common factor among all those I worked with, was the willingness and drive to do more than the rest. They stayed after practice to work on their serve, swing, free kick, or tackle. These athletes didn't need to be told or asked to do this - they were intrinsically motivated to do it themselves. These are the traits of a champion minded athlete.

There are numerous stories of great players who did more to get ahead. Kobe Bryant, the legendary Laker's basketball player, was known to work out at 4:00am. Soccer star Cristiano Ronaldo is known for staying after practice to work on his free kicks and technical skills. Former World Cup rugby stars Dan Carter and Jonny Wilkinson would spend hours alone working on their kicking. Serbian tennis champion

Novak Djokovic hit against the wall for countless hours. Achieving greatness is not a coincidence. The best simply do more. They put in the extra time and they make the extra effort.

Your goals are your own. If being good is good enough, then that's ok - it's your call. But, if you want to be truly exceptional in what you do, then you must put in the extra work. The pain of hard work is nothing compared to the pain of regret. It's your choice - your desire. If your desire is truly to become a champion, do everything you can to improve yourself. Practice hard, refine your skills, study the game, assess your opponents, maximize your strengths and work on your weaknesses, improve your speed, endurance, power, agility, balance, coordination, nutrition, hydration, recovery, and rest. Train mental and emotional toughness. Maintain a positive attitude. Keep learning. When it's all over you'll have no regrets and you'll know you gave it your all. Go the distance.

* * *

*Champions do more. They don't need to be asked.*

# You Get What You Give

*Excellence starts with great effort.*

W hat's the number one regret of athletes who fall short of reaching their goals? Failing to maximize their ability due to lack of effort or commitment. Often when athletes reach the end of their career, they look back and wonder, "What if I had just done a little more, tried just a little bit harder?" Avoid having regrets by consistently giving your best effort.

A great effort stems from a great attitude. Effort is a controllable, a choice you make in each practice, training session, and competition. Giving great effort elicits great results that extend beyond the playing field - to school, to relationships, to work, and to life in general. Nothing great is ever achieved without giving great effort. Champion minded athletes are consistent in the pursuit of greatness, having a great attitude and giving a great effort. The effort you give is directly related to the results you get.

According to Carol Dweck of Stanford University, having a growth mindset is essential to giving great effort. Champion minded athletes understand that mistakes and failures are part of the learning process. They embrace challenges, understanding that failure is an opportunity to learn and to grow. Athletes with a fixed mindset avoid challenges and fear failure, believing that failure defines their ability. Champion minded athletes persist where others give up. The United States Mens' Paralympic Soccer team I began consulting with in 2017 provides a great example. Tragedy has struck many of these men, creating obstacles ranging from brain injuries to strokes, but their belief and "never-say-die" mentalities are truly inspiring and incredible!

When I asked the captain of the team, Kevin Hensley, what being champion minded meant to him, he answered, " It's someone who dedicates him or herself to becoming better everyday. Someone whose teammates can rely on through the good and bad times. They demand the best from themselves and others."

Athletes, do not limit yourselves by avoiding challenges, getting defensive, giving up, lacking effort, ignoring feedback, and feeling threatened by the success of others. Instead, believe that you can always get better by embracing challenges, persisting when faced with setbacks, giving great effort in the pursuit of mastery, accepting and learning from criticism, and finding inspiration in the success of others. Leave no room for regret.

\* \* \*

*It takes ZERO talent to get to practice early or do the extra work required.*

*Talent might make you good, but its your attitude and work ethic that will make you great.*

# Sweep the Sheds

*Champion minded athletes lead by example.*

Champion minded athletes and teams set good examples on and off the field. During the 2016/17 season, after a game against the Philadelphia 76's, Lebron James and Kyrie Irving of the Cavaliers lingered in the locker room to talk to reporters. As Irving addressed the press, James began walking around, not to wait his turn, but to clean up after his teammates who had already left the locker room.

In addition to handing his own laundry bag to the room's attendants, James picked up and delivered another half dozen bags filled with his teammates' dirty clothes. Though the four-time MVP tidied up after his teammates without complaint, he suggested that those who had left their clothes behind might receive a talking-to about general cleanliness. "Hopefully I only have to say something once," James said, "We can't leave the locker room like that." This is a great example of leading by example. James didn't want his team or the franchise to be seen as disrespectful or as a culture with poor standards.

One of the 15 principles of the All Blacks rugby team is "Sweep the Sheds." After each practice or match, the players clean up after themselves. They set an example of personal humility, a cardinal All Blacks value. Each player, no matter what their status, takes responsibility for his own mess. They have a standard - to leave places better than they found them.

Champion minded athletes help build the culture and set the standards for the team. They don't expect it to only come from the coach only. Champion minded athletes lead by example and do not hesitate to call out teammates when necessary to maintain the standards. They believe that even a towel or empty water bottle left on the ground shows poor standards, poor discipline, and a lack of respect for others. They believe that how they are in the small things will be how they are in the big things. This is also how a great culture is built - player to player accountability. The champion minded always aim to leave a great impression wherever they go. They protect their culture, reputation and identity at all times.

* * *

*Culture doesn't change when a coach is the only one holding players accountable. Cultures are built by players holding each other accountable also.*

# Kindness

## *You will always be remembered by how you made others feel.*

No matter how gifted, skilled, or accomplished you may be, you will be remembered by how you made others feel. In the world of top level sports, there are many highly-skilled athletes, some who are famous and wealthy. Even though they might dazzle us with their exceptional skills and abilities, it's their personalities and kindness that touch and impact us most.

Acts of kindness have many forms. As an athlete, helping the coach set up or break down practice equipment is a great way to show kindness. Take time at the end of a competition to thank officials, volunteers, coaches, teammates, and family. American tennis coach and former professional tennis player, Brad Gilbert, made sure his players (including world number ones Andre Agassi and Andy Roddick) thanked all of the tournament staff, ball kids and volunteers before leaving the site!

Any random acts of kindness are welcome. We have seen many great athletes such as Ben Cohen, Lionel Messi, Simone Biles, Tim Tebow, Kevin Anderson, and Roger Federer give their time and efforts to charities and projects that help those less fortunate. Champion minded athletes love giving back. They acknowledge they have been blessed to do what they do in their lives. Not only do acts of kindness help others, but they also increase your own energy and attitude. Developing into a good person is even more important than developing into a good athlete.

## 5 Examples of Acts of Kindness:

1. Thanking parents for all the time spent transporting you to practices and competitions, supporting you, cheering for you, and making the journey possible for you.

2. Treating everyone, regardless of status or position, with the same respect.

3. Thanking coaches, staff, officials, volunteers, fans, drivers, etc.

4. Lending your time (and skills) to a charity organization or foundation.

5. Having empathy for others who are going through tough times (injury, life issues, etc.)

* * *

*No matter how educated, wealthy, accomplished, or talented you are - how you treat people is ultimately what matters.*

# What Image are You Portraying?

*Your reputation is being built everyday.*

A thletes: take a moment to think about how you size-up your opponents.

As you read the names on the draw or entry list, do you think of the strengths and weaknesses they have in their game, of their behavior when they compete, of their general attitude, positive or negative, whether they are tough competitors, fighters or quitters, or whether they play fair or cheat?

When your opponents see your name in the draw or entry list, they do exactly the same thing. You build your reputation everyday. How you act and work at practice, how you interact at social events, on social media, and during competition (including the locker room, restaurants, and hotel), all contribute to the image you display to others. Everyday you are building an image. How you carry yourself, how you treat others (parents, coaches, teammates, opponents, officials), and how you react to adversity send a message about who you are and the standards you keep. Even the way you shake your opponents hand can tell them how confident you are of yourself. What image are you portraying?

To be a champion, one needs to think like a champion, look like a champion, act like a champion, and live like a champion.

\* \* \*

*Everyday you are building an image.*

# Social Media

*Champion minded athletes
are mindful of what they post and share.*

Technology offers quick and easy access to information on just about anything at any time. Social media allows connection to the personal lives of friends, family, acquaintances, people you've never met, celebrities, politicians, and anyone and everyone in between. We can see what they are having for dinner, where they go on vacation, their pets, work outs at the gym, shopping outings, engagements, anything from the mundane to the incredibly intimate.

Athletes: it's important to understand that just as you search and gather information about other people, parents, coaches, schools, businesses, and employers, they may be searching, accessing information, and making judgements about you.

What do your posts reveal about you - your character, your lifestyle, your commitment to academic and athletic pursuits, your attitude, your family, your friends, how you spend your time? The list goes on and on. Before you post anything, first think to yourself: is this true? is this helpful? is this inspiring? is this necessary? is this kind? is this respectful? Avoid arguments and debates. Don't use profanity. Don't post pictures you wouldn't want your family, coaches, teachers, bosses or employers to see. Champion minded athletes are careful with what they post and share on social media. Athletes: beware when it comes to your social media. Scholarships, professional contracts, and jobs can be lost, relationships can be damaged, reputations can be ruined, all from one post

Clemson men's soccer head coach, Mike Noonan said that by checking out their social media posts, his coaching staff finds out about a player's character, outlook on life, and personality. He went further saying, "If someone is being critical of a teammate, coach, referee, or situation on social media, that may be suggesting some potential problems down the road."

Athletes: When it comes to social media, pause and think before you post. Don't let a Facebook or Twitter rant cost you the chance of a lucrative contract, college scholarship or job opportunity!

\* \* \*

*Think before you post on social media.*
*Ask yourself: Will this help or hurt my reputation?*

# Failing vs Failure

*Failing and failure are not the same;*
*there's a big difference.*

There's a big difference between failure and failing. Failing is an opportunity to learn and to grow. Unfortunately, many people have a negative view of failing, which prohibits them from learning valuable lessons. Failing is not the opposite of success, it's part of the process to achieve success. Champion minded athletes learn more from their losses than they do from their wins.

Failure is quitting, and there is nothing worse. Quitters are afraid of failing. Quitters seek perfection, which is unattainable and therefore leads to failure.

Making mistakes and failing provides you with valuable feedback to help you make changes for the better. Former world number 1 tennis player, Andy Murray once said, "I'm not afraid of failing. I'm failing all the time."

Winners are not afraid of losing. Losers are. Failing is part of the process of success. People who avoid failing also avoid success. Champion minded athletes seek excellence, which requires failing and trying again.

## 5 Ways Champion Minded People View Failing:

1. Champion minded people are often industry leaders, yet they still make mistakes. They understand that failing is part of success, so they are not afraid to fail or to look foolish.

2. Champion minded people have a different perspective of failing. They have a growth mindset and they view challenges as opportunities to learn.

3. Champion minded people view failing as an opportunity to try again and to achieve better results.

4. Champion minded people understand there will be obstacles and challenges along the path to success. They face them and embrace them.

5. Champion minded people know that every time they make a mistake, they are learning.

\* \* \*

*Failing is an opportunity to learn and to grow.*

# Practice:
# Constructive & Affirmative

*One breaks you down, the other builds you up.*

Athletes: it's important to understand the different types of practices which help you prepare to compete. During earlier preparation, practices should focus on specific technical, tactical, physical, mental, and emotional goals. These workouts should challenge, push, and motivate you to perform. There will be lots of feedback - some you may not want to hear. These practices can be "ugly." We apply the term "ugly" because it represents the realities of competition in a practice setting. Be prepared to push your limit in constructive practices. They prepare you to handle those tests when you compete. You must be tested and have to problem-solve in practice to be prepared to do so when it counts. These practices are constructive and vitally important, but they are not always fun. Athletes confront their monkeys so that the gorillas don't show up come competition time!

If earlier preparation practices test you and push you, the practices leading up to competition are meant to relax you and to build you up. In the final few days before competing, no significant changes should be made technically or physically - there's just not enough time to consolidate them. You can't "cram" for competition. You're either prepared or you're not. The days right before competition are not the time to panic and to frantically try to force last minute fixes, changes, or additions to your game. The practices right before competition should be positive. They should highlight your strengths. They should be relaxed, fun, and free of stress. These practices focus on nurturing a confident mindset, and developing a calm resolve. Athletes - approach these practices leading up to competition positively, enjoying your favorite shots and patterns of play. Perform your calming rituals, and enjoy yourself. This is the time for hopeful determination, for inspired and courageous self-belief. You're confident and ready.

When observing practice sessions at professional sports events, the differences between the experienced, established champions and the lower ranked contenders is striking. Watching Usain Bolt, Roger Federer, or the All Blacks practicing a day or two out before competing, they always seem to be enjoying themselves, engaging with the fans and often with the media. They understand that the work has been done already, so it's time to enjoy the occasion and the thrill of competing.

\* \* \*

*You're either prepared or not.*
*Put worry aside and just compete.*

M

# Normal Doesn't Create Excellence

*Champion minded athletes are not "normal."*

It's not normal to stand on the Olympic podium with a medal around your neck. It's not normal to win Wimbledon or the Super Bowl or the World Series or the Stanley Cup or The Masters. To reach the highest levels of sport requires a certain level of *not-normal*. Champion minded athletes make choices which may appear to others as a little bit crazy. People will say "you're obsessed, you're not normal!" and they're right, because reaching the elite level of athletics is not a normal journey.

After a training session in Copenhagen, Denmark, I remember chatting with Scott Evans over a cup of coffee. A three time Olympian in Badminton, the fiercely driven Irishman told me, "It's not a normal life - It can't be. I'm addicted to it, and want to get better everyday."

It's not normal to do thousands upon thousands of repetitions to master a skill, or, through all the hours of training, to inflict pain and soreness on your body. This is why greatness is not for everyone.

When Kobe Bryant was on stage accepting the Icon Award at the ESPYs, he said:

> We're not on this stage just because of talent
> or ability. We're up here because of 4 a.m.
> We're up here because of two-a-days or five-
> a-days. We're up here because we had a

*dream and let nothing stand in our way. If anything tried to bring us down, we used it to make us stronger.*

I've been blessed to train and work with many elite athletes - world champions, world number 1's, and Olympians. They are a little weird and different in their own special ways. As stated, they aren't normal. In my first book, *7 Keys to Being a Great Coach,* I wrote that "normal doesn't create excellence." It never will. In fact, one of the commonalities of all the champion performers is that they have borderline psychosis and an obsession with being the best at what they do. They fear normal because they want to be exceptional.

\* \* \*

*"Today, I will do what others won't, so tomorrow I can do what others can't."*

- Jerry Rice

*The champion minded*
*are prepared to do what others aren't*
*prepared to do.*
*They are obsessed with improving.*

# Excellence Is Not For Everyone

## *Rise above mediocrity.*

The very fact that you are reading this book tells me something about you. It tells me you want to get the very best from yourself everyday. If you're aiming for greatness as an athlete (or in life), then be prepared to be misunderstood, ridiculed, labeled as weird, strange, sometimes unsociable, and selfish. Along the journey, you also better be prepared to lose some people who you might have thought were your friends. When aiming for greatness, there will be imbalances in your life. Yes, you're not normal!

It's a choice. You can choose to be disciplined, wake up early, work hard, put in the extra effort or you can just stay average. Be sure that your choices reflect your goals. If you say that it is your goal to be a collegiate or professional athlete but your choices are not aligned with that goal, it's not going to happen. Talent might be the entry ticket, but the attitude and work ethic you bring everyday are the traits that will make you great.

When you strive for excellence, there will be people who will attempt to hold you back. Don't compromise your standards to accommodate them. Mediocrity exists inside your comfort zone. To break away from mediocrity, you'll have to get outside of your comfort zone, to look and act differently from those you leave behind. Don't look back! Surround yourself with like-minded people who share your high standards and values. Surround yourself with greatness everyday.

Distance yourself from those who hold you back. Let's be clear - those who choose to be average are not necessarily bad people. They may simply have different dreams and goals. Not everyone aspires to be great, and that is just fine, as long as they do not try to hold you back or to impede your progress.

Don't be afraid to fail or to make mistakes. Only through trying and failing, and trying again can you get better. You can achieve the extraordinary. Rise above mediocrity to pursue greatness. Remember that excellence is not for everyone. It is only for those who are willing to give their very best.

* * *

*Never lower your standards for someone else.*
*Rather let them rise up to yours.*

# Choice vs Sacrifice

*Sacrifice is reactive. Choice is proactive.*

I've watched numerous interviews and read many articles in which an athlete says that they made many sacrifices to get to where they are now.

When you pursue your passion, your purpose, your goals, it's not a sacrifice, it's a choice you make. Making a healthy choice at mealtime is not a sacrifice, it is a decision. Deciding to go home and get enough sleep instead of staying out late and socializing is not a sacrifice, it is a choice. These are choices you make for yourself. If you would rather stay up late at a friend's birthday party the night before a competition - go for it! But, don't be surprised if you're not pleased with your performance the next day. When asked by a friend why he didn't attend many parties, former NBA star player Kevin Johnson said: "Parties won't take me to where I want to go." It's your choice. Only you are responsible for your choices. Take ownership of your choices.

If someone else (coach, trainer, parent, teammate, etc.) is pressuring you to make choices you do not want to make, then the goal is out of focus. Your support system and your entourage should be aware of your goals and should help you make decisions according to your goals. If other people want the goal more than you do, it's their goal, not yours. Sacrifice is defined as something of value given up for the sake of something else. Synonyms include: surrender, forfeiture, abandonment, and resignation. None of those words are positive affirmations of a personal decision.

Choice is defined as an act of selecting or making a decision when faced with two or more possibilities. Synonyms include: option, selection, preference, and pick. A choice is a positive action. Pursuing your vision, chasing your dream, and achieving your goal are choices only you can make. Where others see sacrifices, the champion minded make choices.

* * *

*Champion minded athletes don't believe in making sacrifices. Instead, they believe in making choices - choices that take them to where they aspire to be.*

# Work Smarter, Not Harder

*Champion minded athletes engage in specific, purposeful training.*

Quantity does not equal quality. Too much of a good thing can become a bad thing. I've seen athletes waste good intentions and energy on drills or exercises that really do not have any useful impact on their development. It becomes just stuff to do - busywork. Doing the work just to log the hours is not beneficial to the specific goals required for each sport. Yes, it takes extra work to gain the slight edge. However, it must be specific and purposeful work.

Sometimes, it's good to hit pause and ask yourself whether the work you are doing is making you better or just making you tired?

What's better - 20 hours a week at 50% or 10 hours a week at 100%? The latter of course. Consider the intensity and the extra time needed to rest! I can't tell you how often I witness young athletes logging senseless hours when they could be spending their time better by getting more recovery and more rest. Remember, the amount of time spent does not indicate how hard you are working.

Athletes - identify the specific areas in which you need to improve and train accordingly. Put your energy into what you need to do to improve and not just into what you like to do. Have priorities to your training and don't simply fill time to be busy.

Continually assess and ask yourself why you are training the way you are training. Make it your mission to understand the purpose behind each and everything you do. Save your time and energy for what really matters.

\* \* \*

*We achieve more when we chase the vision instead of the competition.*

# The Best Are Obsessed

*The champion minded have great desire.*

It's Christmas morning 2016. I've just returned home from Delray beach where I took one of my visiting athletes through a grueling sand session. I call it the "Christmas cracker." Some may call it extreme, but to be a champion, no matter what day it is, the work still needs to be done. Growing up, I was so determined to become the best athlete, I felt those "vacation days" were the ones where I could get an edge on my opponents - physically and mentally.

Over the years, I've learned that the best of the best are deeply obsessed with getting better. When it comes to putting in the required work, they have a totally different relationship with effort. They don't make excuses and they don't have time for people who make them either. They are on a different mission than the rest - a mission to succeed.

I'm often asked what separates the good from the great athletes. My answer? Certainly, it's the athlete's coachability, their bigger purpose, and their work ethic. But, the most important one is their obsession for succeeding.

Former Liverpool and England soccer captain, Steven Gerrard, said it best,

> *I was obsessed. Obsessed with being the best player in training every single day, and if I wasn't, I'd go home and think about it and try and do it again the next day. When you get that sniff and that little bit of hope, you've got*

*to be obsessed to move them (teammates) out*
*of the way. You have to be obsessed.*

When I asked my good friend, Michael Beale, who was the assistant coach at Sao Paulo football club in Brazil (also formerly at Liverpool and Chelsea), about what he saw in the best young players he'd worked with, he responded, "The best ones are obsessive about improving themselves. Especially when learning a new technique, they will become obsessive about mastering it."

As I'm writing this, (it's Christmas Day, remember!), I'm on Twitter, and an Australian female Olympian track runner I follow, just tweeted: "Christmas day and got my 21km (13.1mile) run in before 7:00am."

\* \* \*

### *"You have to be obsessed."*

- Steven Gerrard

*"This is an obsession. Talent does not exist, we are all equals as human beings. You could be anyone if you put in the time. You will reach the top, and that's that. I am not talented. I am obsessed."*

- Conor McGregor

# Learn To Say No

*Champion minded athletes know how and when to say no.*

Champion minded athletes protect their health and wellness. This means knowing how and when to say no. Saying no is not selfish. Saying no requires wisdom and skill and may, at times, be painful. Many times, during interviews, elite athletes speak about the sacrifices they have made along the way to be where they are now. Sacrifice is defined as an act of giving up something valued for the sake of something else regarded as more important. This is a choice. If your goal truly is to be an elite athlete, there will be sacrifices along the way. I'm not a huge fan of the word sacrifice. The choices you make along your journey reflect your commitment to your vision and your goals.

There will be social events that you don't want to miss. There will be times when "being normal" seems so appealing. Understand that you are on a different path by your own choosing. Champion minded athletes have different priorities and standards, which can make for some difficult decisions. This doesn't mean that you will not have friends or fun or a social life. Remember your long-term goal and vision. There's plenty of fun to be had - it just may have to wait awhile (delayed gratification versus instant gratification).

It's important to give back. Make time to mentor younger, less experienced athletes. Choose the charities and/or causes you support and commit to them. If your schedule allows you to give extra, that's great, but be careful what you commit your time and energy to. Always be conscious of your energy as giving too much leaves you with nothing left to give. As selfish as it sounds, you come first.

Surround yourself with people who understand and support your long-term goals. They will help you make the tough decisions with your best interests at heart. Avoid those who tempt you to abandon your discipline. Avoid those who ask for so much that agreeing to help would compromise your journey to reach your goal. Learn how and when to say no. Protect your health and wellness to stay on track with your long-term goals.

* * *

*Your commitment to your vision and goals are reflected in the choices you make along your journey.*

# SECTION 5:

# *Before Competition*

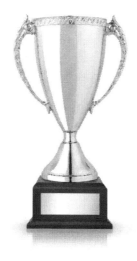

# A Fundamental Approach

## *Prepare To Win.*

1. Build a structure to your day with routines, as this creates positive and winning habits.

2. Aim for between 7-9 hours of sleep per night.

3. Have a set bedtime and a set wake up time.

4. Hydrate consistently throughout day, sipping at least every 15-20 minutes.

5. Have a good breakfast. Good choices include: oatmeal, egg whites, whole wheat bread, and fruit.

6. Try to include at least 10-15g of protein with every meal.

7. Snack consistently throughout the day. Don't go without nutrition for more than 90 minutes.

8. For 20 minutes each day, read something inspiring.

9. For 20 – 30 minutes each day (preferably after lunch), take a nap.

10. Stretch and foam roll every 12 hours (once in the morning and again in the evening).

11. Before bedtime, consume 10g of protein.

12. In order to perform optimally when practicing or competing; bring enough food, drinks, and items to meet your individual needs.

13. Plan ahead. Give yourself plenty of travel time. Make it a habit to arrive 10 minutes early.

14. Get up early and make your bed each morning – this is your first disciplined act of the day.

15. Properly preparing gives you your best chance to start the morning off great. Pack your bag and prepare your drinks and snacks the night before practice or competition.

\* \* \*

*"Preparation can be defined in three words:*
*Leave. Nothing. Undone."*

- George Allen

# Find Your Purpose

*Passion isn't enough;*
*you need purpose to succeed.*

Y ou've most likely heard the saying, "Follow your passion." I've discovered passion is not enough to achieve what really matters in life. To achieve happiness, contentment and fulfillment, you need to have a deeper purpose.

What's the difference between the two? Passion is the compelling emotions behind your dreams. It's what you find stimulating and fun to do. It's your feelings that drive your passion. Purpose, on the other hand, is the *why* behind it all - your deeper, inner reason.

Mark Twain once said, "the two greatest days of your life are the day you were born, and the day you find out what your purpose is." If you don't know what your purpose is, then you don't know why you are here, and sometimes it can be hard to keep going.

When I sit down with a new athlete or a client, one of the first questions I like to ask them is, "What is your purpose?" At first they'll look at me a little startled, and then proceed to answer the question with something related to their line of work or chosen sport. But that's not what I'm looking for.

I posed this exact question to an Olympic athlete I consulted with before the 2012 London Olympics. She'd been finding it difficult to motivate herself. A few years prior, she'd dealt with depression. Answering my question, she told me her purpose was to win a medal. "Fair enough", I said, "but that's a goal." I wanted to know her life's purpose. She went away and thought about it, and then came back the next week with this answer: "My deeper purpose is to be able to inspire people who are going through what I did, so that they too can overcome whatever challenges they have going on in their lives." A few weeks later, we met again, and I noticed something totally different in her. She had more motivation and assuredness about her. She told me that in finding her deeper purpose, her ability to train longer and harder had increased. She now had a deeper purpose and not just a passing goal. She even said that after her career was done on the track, she wanted to get involved in setting up a foundation to help others who suffered from the same condition.

During Mark Zuckerberg's commencement address at Harvard in May 2017, the Facebook founder commented, "Purpose is that sense that we are part of something bigger than ourselves, that we are needed, that we have something better ahead to work for. Purpose is what creates true happiness."

The champion minded understand that it's their purpose in life that matters most.

\* \* \*

*Purpose is an incredible alarm clock.*

# How the Champion Minded Compete

*Champion minded athletes
are 100% committed to the process.*

W hen the champion minded compete, they are 100% committed to the process. They are completely present and focused in the moment because they understand this is what gives them the best chance to succeed. They don't dwell in the past. They don't worry about the future. They think and act in the moment.

The champion minded play freely and fearlessly. They have learned that playing with an outcome-based mindset impedes "freeness" and only attracts fear.

The champion minded compete hard all the time. Regardless of the opposition, they are always 100% committed to preparing and giving their best effort.

No matter the score or the odds, the champion minded always believe they can succeed. They maintain helpful self-talk and habits even in the midst of adversity. They know that if they are 100% committed to competing, there is no time for complaining.

They hustle. They fight. They never let up. They are relentless. They give nothing away. They display no negativity or poor body language, because they know it gives their opponents hope. They are 100% focused on the controllables.

The champion minded judge themselves on the effort and commitment they give, not on what they get.

*The champion minded are always 100% committed to preparing and giving their best effort.*

# 5000-1 Odds

*Champion minded athletes*
*always believe they have a chance.*

You don't have to follow soccer to appreciate what English team Leicester City Football Club accomplished in the 2015-2016 season. Leicester City's championship is the most unlikely victory in sports history. For Leicester City to win the title, bookmakers in the UK set the pre-season odds at 5,000-1. At the time, other 5,000-1 odds were available for Elvis Presley to be found alive and for Barack Obama to play cricket for England!

Leicester City Football Club, also known as the Foxes, had slipped to the bottom of the Premier League in the 2014-2015 season and faced certain relegation. Incredibly, they won 7 of their last 9 matches to survive dropping down. Described as one of the Premier League's greatest ever escapes from relegation, their upturn gained international attention. Just five games into the next season, coach Nigel Pearson was sacked and former Chelsea manager Claudio Ranieri was appointed as the new manager. Against tremendous odds, Leicester City won the 2015-2016 Premier League, their first top-level football championship. Their title win is widely regarded as one of the greatest upsets in sports history.

The message here is a simple one. Ignore the critics and focus on the process. Even when others don't, champion minded athletes believe in themselves, in their teammates and in the process. They focus on what they can control. They don't let a history of results nor the opinions and criticisms of others get them down. They focus on their own journey. They believe that the impossible is always possible.

## Other long-shot victories of note:

- 1,000-1: 1980 US Men's Hockey Olympic Gold
- 1,000-1: 2013 Auburn football National Championship
- 999-1: 2011 St. Louis Cardinals World Series
- 500-1: 1987 Minnesota Twins World Series
- 300-1: 1999 St. Louis Rams Super Bowl

\* \* \*

*No matter what the odds are against you, remember there's always a chance!*

# There Are No Secrets

*Put in the work and stay disciplined.*

After lifting his sixth PSA Squash World Tour title in a row at the 2017 Bellevue Squash Classic, Frenchman Greg Gaultier returned to the top of the World Rankings to break his own record as the oldest-ever World No.1.

Having previously worked with a couple of the world's top players in the past, I always admired Greg from a distance. He had an unparalleled desire, attitude and work ethic to be the best he could be.

For those of you who are unfamiliar with the game of Squash, it is without a doubt, one of the most physically demanding sports there is. It is brutal!

A few days after he reached this milestone, I sent Greg a text message to congratulate him. I also asked him his secret to staying motivated and how he dealt with the tougher times during his career.

Greg replied, "Well first, you always need targets. With no targets, there is no motivation. At this stage, as I'm getting towards the end of my playing career, I have more short-term targets than long-term ones."

When questioned about how he'd dealt with the failures and the lows in his career, he explained, "You have to take it on the chin and stand up to those defeats, not run away with easy excuses or blame others. It's always good to analyze the good and the bad. It's about persevering in your daily work and believing you can."

Finally, Greg went on to say that there were no secrets. It all came down to putting in the hard work, being disciplined, persevering and believing. He also mentioned the importance of surrounding yourself with a good team that you can trust and with whom you can communicate. Wise words from a master of his trade and a perfect example of a champion minded athlete.

* * *

*"It's about persevering in your daily work and believing you can."*

- Greg Gaultier

# Control the Controllables

*Let go of what you have no control over.*

Discovering serenity changed my own personal journey. I wish I had caught on to this when competing as a kid. Serenity is the state of being calm, peaceful, and untroubled. Having serenity includes having the wisdom to know the difference between what can and cannot be changed or controlled.

Champion minded athletes possess serenity. They focus on what is within their control and what is beyond their control neither distracts nor distresses them. A few years ago I worked with the former South African cricket captain, Graeme Smith. The South African team had just returned from the subcontinent after a tough tour against a strong Indian team. Tricky pitches, extreme humidity, and raucous crowds make for difficult playing conditions. I asked Graeme about how they were able to play and focus amid these formidable challenges. He answered that they chose to focus on what they could control and didn't let the things beyond their control get in the way. Each athlete has limited physical, mental, and emotional energy. Stressing and worrying about things beyond your control only rob you of your energy.

## Controllables:

- Preparation
- Routines
- Effort & Attitude
- Body Language
- Reaction to mistakes/bad calls
- Energy
- Self-talk

## Uncontrollables:

- Quality of Playing Surface
- Weather
- Umpire/Referee/Official Calls
- Opponent Performance or Behavior (gamesmanship, cheating, trash talk, disrespect)
- Outcome/Result
- Spectators' Behavior

\* \* \*

*Focus on what you can control.*
*Let go of what you can't.*

# Energy

*Champion minded athletes
and teams have a great energy.*

Teams and individuals, who consistently produce winning results, have a great energy and aura. They exude confidence and positivity. Their posture and body language, along with their interpersonal communications, project poise and a calm assuredness. Your body language communicates a powerful message to those around you, especially to your opponents.

At the world championship or Olympic level, I enjoy watching volleyball. Following a mistake or a lost point, teammates encourage each other with enthusiastic sincerity and celebrate each other with genuine passion following triumph. Champion minded teams and athletes understand the importance of projecting great energy whether facing victory or defeat.

Athletes, if I were to show up to your match already underway, would I be able to know who was winning and losing by what energy was being displayed through body language and interpersonal communications? I hope to see both teams or athletes looking positively energized and giving full effort to competition. Usually, I don't need to look at the scoreboard to know who is winning or losing. All I have to do is to observe the body language and the competitors' energy.

Remember, you are either giving away energy to your opponents through negative body language and emotions, or you are gaining more of it by staying positive, engaged, and excited.

When you compete, bring a champion attitude and confident body language.

\* \* \*

*Your energy is everything!*

# Focus in the Moment

*Champion minded athletes don't dwell on the past or worry about the future, they focus in the present moment.*

A penalty kick, free-throw, second serve, putt, or a field goal, which would be routine under normal circumstances may become overwhelmingly challenging under pressure. Athletes: have you experienced this? A shot that you've successfully performed countless times misses the mark during a pressure-filled moment of competition. Given an athlete's skills and experience in a stressful situation, this reaction is usually linked to choking or underperforming.

Why do athletes choke? It is a loss of focus in the present moment. The shift in focus away from the present goes in two directions - past and future. Dwelling on a past bad play or a missed opportunity, keeps the athlete's mind from focusing on the present moment. Fear or excitement about the outcome - winning or losing - also steals focus away from the present moment. Both emotions are crippling. In either case, players either freeze up, play it too safely, or become overly aggressive - they lose mental focus and physical control.

Training under stress is vitally important. Practicing your responses to pressure will help you to stay calm when it counts. Follow a ritual. Repeat a mantra to yourself. Let go of the past. Don't get ahead of yourself. These habits will help you stay focused in the moment.

At the 2016 British Open, Phil Mickelson and Henrik Stenson completely distanced themselves from the rest of the field and matched each other nearly shot for shot. On the final Sunday, the stakes could not have been higher  Stenson shot a final round of 63 for 264, a record 20-under par, three strokes ahead of runner-up and 2013 Champion, Mickelson. Stenson credited the win to staying calm, sticking to the process, and not getting ahead of himself.

When 2010 winning Alabama Quarterback Greg McElroy stepped to the line of scrimmage for the first play of the biggest game of his life, he was 100% focused on the process. He said: "Every play is a new beginning and has nothing to do with the last play. If I did something boneheaded or brilliant, [each new play] was still a chance to start over."

By focusing only on what he could do in the moment—not what had already happened, or what he had to accomplish over the coming hours—he kept his nerve and helped his team to 37-10 win.

\* \* \*

*The champion minded athletes stay in the moment.*

*The champion minded
have a short-term memory.
They're able to forget a bad play and
move on quickly with a great attitude.*

# Normal is Easy.
# Excellence is Hard.

*Never apologize for having high standards.*

If you want to do great things, you need to be willing to be different. Most people do not choose the path to becoming a champion. Most are simply not willing to make the commitments and choices involved. The path to excellence comes with a price - early mornings, time away from friends and family, missed holiday celebrations, a sore and fatigued body, and nutrition and hydration restrictions just to name a few. When you decide to take the path to excellence, prepare to be ridiculed. Understand that excellence always threatens mediocrity. Mediocre people hate hard work. When you choose excellence, expect to be labeled as strange, obsessed, and unsociable. The choices you make on the way to greatness will not always be popular. Expect to be criticized and misunderstood.

That's why it's important to surround yourself with people that reflect who you want to be and how you want to feel, people who understand your journey, your lifestyle and your mindset. Those who really want to be in your life will rise up to meet your standards.

Normal is easy. Excellence is hard. Never apologize for having high standards.

Past success does not determine future success. The best performers commit to continually improving themselves. If you want to win consistently, you have to continually improve.

The path to excellence is not easy, but with a positive attitude and mindset, and surrounded by the right people, you can do it! Normal is doing what the rest do. The champion minded strive for excellence.

\* \* \*

*"You have to be odd to be number one."*

- Dr. Seuss

*Not everyone will agree or go along with the higher standards and discipline you've created. But then again, excellence isn't for everyone.*

# Study Your Opponent

*Champion minded athletes
observe and gather information.*

Apolo Ohno is a retired American short track speed skating competitor and an eight-time medalist in the Winter Olympics. He was a scholar of his sport and a legend. Ohno obsessively studied his opponents, watching their behavior, their attitude, their body language, and their interactions with their team and others, etc. He wanted to know their game skills, their strengths and weaknesses, how they handled pressure, if they looked focused or not, and what they did to prepare. When he was at competitions, he would always identify who he would have to be wary of competing against. Ohno said knowing his opponents on and off the track gave him a distinct advantage when it came to competition.

Today, it amazes me how many athletes and players know so little about their opponents. They go to a competition, they compete, and then they go home. Some feel it's their coaches' responsibility to always do the scouting. The champion minded know their opponents. They scout them at tournaments, in the gym, at practice - everywhere! They keep a little book with notes about their opponents. They know their strengths and weaknesses, their breaking points, and their habits.

Athletes: raise your awareness about your opponents. Look for clues - verbal and nonverbal - as you scout your opponents. Watch them compete. Make notes on what you see, because there is a good chance you will come up against them one day.

Scouting is part of a champion minded athlete's preparation. They prepare for their own game, and for their opponent's game.

\* \* \*

*Scouting your opponents is an important part of preparation; the more you know, the better prepared you are to face them.*

# Getting Past Perfectionism

*Champion minded athletes*
*aspire to be the best they can be.*

Athletes - rather than shoot for perfection, aspire to be the best you can be. Aspiring for perfection actually decreases confidence and impedes progress. Champion minded athletes hold themselves accountable to the pursuit of excellence and to incredibly high standards, but not to perfection. These high performers are driven to be the best they can be, but their response to mistakes and failures is a trait which distinguishes champion minded athletes from the rest.

A perfectionist cannot accept a less than perfect performance, which inevitably leads to disappointment, frustration, and discouragement. Champion minded athletes understand that there will be times when they are underperforming. But, despite their less-than-perfect performance, they can fight on. Have you ever surprised yourself with a great shot, only to fail trying to replicate it? Avoid the pitfall of trying to repeat a great performance. Just aim to do the best you can each day.

Perfectionism steals enjoyment and satisfaction from sport. Be aware of expectation, and aim for the best outcome, but be willing and prepared to work through imperfect circumstances. Fiercely determined to succeed, the champion minded athlete abandons the quest for perfection and accepts imperfection. Accepting imperfection does not mean lowering standards. It is accepting the reality that perfection is unattainable. Champion minded athletes always give their best effort, knowing that their best effort will not always equate to their best performance.

\* \* \*

*Instead of aiming for a perfect practice,
aim for a perfect effort.*

# Expectations

*Expectations create unnecessary pressure.*

W hen it comes to the athlete or the team, expectations can be dangerous. Having worked with many elite athletes and teams in a variety of sports, I've seen expectations impede performances and outcomes.

What is expectation?

The Oxford Dictionary states Expectation (def): *a strong belief that something will happen or be the case.* This definition sums up how expectation can increase the pressure on the athlete. The phrase "strong belief" suggests that the person with this strong belief is convinced what they are believing is going to happen. By doing this, they increase the pressure they place on themselves.

When it comes to other people, we need to remember that expectations are only an opinion. For example, we often hear about a certain player or a team who is expected to beat their opponent. But, we know that sports are also about uncontrollables. We can't control what's going happen.

Expectation is also the reason why some athletes let negative emotions get in the way of their performance. This negativity tends to occur when the athlete has anticipated a favorable result, but then begins to panic or to lose control of their focus when it's not going the way they anticipated. Imagine a golfer who felt he could shoot a below par round, but suddenly finds himself five over par.

When expectation gets in the way of performance, the athlete can become frustrated, or even embarrassed, especially when loved ones or supporters are present. These expectations also explain why some athletes can perform even better when loved ones or supporters are not nearby.

So what is the solution? First, replace expectations with "process goals." Take care of what needs to be done in this moment and do it to the best of your ability. Build rituals into your game. Rituals keep you focused on the process.

Your expectations should not be fixed to an outcome or result. Instead, fix them to your process, giving your best effort, and keeping your mind in the present. This is how you learn to perform with confidence!

*  *  *

*Don't let expectations get in the way of sticking to the process.*

# Let go!

## *Caring too much can sometimes impede your performance.*

I've found that when an athlete cares too much (yes, cares to much!) it can impede their ability to perform. They want to succeed so badly they begin to force it, become impatient, and even to begin to beat themselves up!

Caring too much can actually limit performance and put extra pressure on the athlete. The key is to find the balance between caring and letting go. When I refer to letting go, that doesn't mean quitting or giving a lesser effort. It means letting go of expectations and worries about final outcomes.

How often have you witnessed a player trying so damn hard, but things just seem to get worse and worse? Perhaps you've even experienced this yourself. Usually you will find that you've blocked your flow passage. You've become anxious and you've begun to tighten up physically and mentally. You have gone from a flow state to a freeze state.

Pause for a moment and think about when you are just practicing and there's nothing on the line. How do you feel? Happy, free, and relaxed, right? You are freely hitting, swinging, or throwing without a care in the world, and it just feels amazing! You're not concerned about messing up!

Athletes: the next time you are feeling off, or you find that the harder you are trying the worse things become, pause for a moment, relax your breathing, and try to free yourself up by caring less, taking a step back, and letting go a bit. In the end, it's the overthinking which hurts you. Stop it! Instead, use strategies like humor, positive self-talk, or giving yourself a free pass to make some mistakes.

Sometimes you just have to let go, and let things be what they are. Trust in your preparation and don't force it. When you let go of expectations and free your mind, you will start to play well again.

* * *

*Caring too much is one of the biggest reasons why athletes fail to produce their optimum performance.*

*Make sure its your mind that's in control, and not your emotions.*

# Always Compete

*Do you demand the best from yourself?*

Athletes: no one will *give* you starting positions, games, titles, and championships. At the top of the game, there are no freebies. The same rule applies in life - you have to work for what you want! When recruiting or having try-outs, coaches consider the intangibles (character, leadership, coachable-ness, etc.). Coaches aren't just looking for talent, they are looking for tough competitors! Legendary Tennessee women's basketball coach, Pat Summitt, says, "I look for competitors when I am recruiting. I look for players from winning programs because I know they've been in competitive situations, and they've won and they understand how to win."

Athletes: in practice, are you pushing yourself to your limits? Do you demand the best of yourself? In order to surpass your previous limits and expectations, be willing to be uncomfortable. In order to improve, you have to be driven. The way you practice will be the way you compete. To become a better competitor practice your physical, mental, and emotional toughness.

While I was chatting with Paige Williams, a member of the England ladies u/23 international football team, she told me, "I like to push myself during practice. I have always been about getting uncomfortable, because that's where we grow most." Having just defeated Sweden with the England team, Paige went on to say, "I love to compete, even in practice I want to win."

Champion minded athletes compete during practice. Athletes: compete with yourself. Compete with your teammates. This will raise the intensity level during practice and you'll be better prepared for competition. Being soft on your teammates does them a disservice. Pushing them will only make them better.

American swimmer and Olympic gold medalist Conor Dwyer says that during practice he competes against his teammates just like it's a race. "It's a win-win situation", he said. "You push me, I'll push you, and we both improve."

On many occasions, I have witnessed less talented athletes succeed simply because they brought a better attitude and greater, more determined effort. Champion minded athletes understand that the way they practice (physically, mentally, and emotionally), will become the way they compete. You will never meet a tough competitor who practices easy.

* * *

*"Even in practice I refuse to lose."*

- Conor Dwyer

*When you have consistently practiced and developed the right routines, it takes you from a thinking mode to a trusting and instinctive mode.*

# The Importance of Winning Self-Talk

*Champion minded athletes
build their confidence through self-talk.*

E lite athletes recognize that confidence is a key factor to peak performance. An athlete brimming with confidence has fully prepared for competition and possesses self-belief. Self-belief stems from a positive attitude and self-talk.

Athletes: you can talk yourself into and out of just about anything! In order to be successful, you need to be your own biggest motivator. Your inner voice needs to speak encouragement, support, comfort, hope, and strength. Managing your self-talk can be incredibly difficult, but the ability to control what you say to yourself is an incredibly important skill in sport and in life. Remember, just like any other skill, positive self-talk is trainable.

If you have negative self-talk in practice, you'll have negative self-talk in competition. Negativity leads to choking, panic, hopelessness, fear, anxiety, nervousness, worry, tension, and doubt. Negativity clings to past frustration, disappointment, and defeat, which leads to a fatalistic, critical, defeatist, and pessimistic view of the future.

Having positive self-talk in practice will translate to positive self-talk in competition. Positivity exists in the present moment, letting go of the past, and remaining hopefully expectant of the future. Rather than dwelling on past results that cannot be changed or future outcomes that have not yet happened, staying positive in the present moment keeps athletes focused on the task at hand.

It's unrealistic to think negative thoughts and responses will never happen. When you display negativity, it boosts your opponent's energy and gives them hope and belief. Champion minded athletes dismiss negative emotions quickly and replace them with positive responses. While negative self-talk and defeated body language are self-sabotaging habits, positive self-talk and confident body language are self-affirming habits.

* * *

*You can talk yourself into and out of*
*just about anything!*

# J2

*Have a clear objective and vision in practice and competition.*

A s a coach, I try to keep things simple. J2 is an abbreviation for "just two," which is a coaching method I use when I'm training my athletes. Instructions should be clear and messages concise. Athletes - identify the main ideas your coach is trying to convey to you (good coaches make this easy). Practices should follow an outline and have a theme for each session. It should be easy to follow the progression and to grasp the main idea.

Over-coaching is a common occurrence - this does not mean they are not good coaches, but if you find yourself feeling overloaded with more information than is possible to process at the given moment, or if you find yourself zoning-out during lengthy explanations and instructions, challenge yourself to find the main ideas and the purpose behind each drill or exercise. Practices should be structured around a clearly and concisely stated purpose.

When you practice on your own, you have the freedom to choose what you want to focus on! Choose one or two main objectives (technical and/or tactical), and build your drills and exercises around those areas of focus. Don't try to do too much.

J2 also applies to pre-competition. Approach each match with a clear plan. Competition objectives should primarily be tactical. Match time is not the time to focus on technique. Competition elevates pressure and stress-levels, so goals and instructions need to be simple and as clear as possible. Keeping notes, and going to your notes during play, is helpful. Keep your notes short and to the point. Even a single key word or a short phrase can be helpful reminders to stay focused. Over-analyzing is physically and mentally paralyzing. Have a plan and be prepared to adapt as the situation evolves.

\* \* \*

*When it comes to practice, keep it simple and focus on no more than two priorities for each session.*

# Pre-Competition Routines

*Champion minded athletes
have consistent and complete preparation.*

Before competing, elite athletes have routines and rituals they consistently perform. Common routines include arrival time at the venue, what and when they eat prior to play, choice of pre-game music, etc. These routines help the athlete be mentally, physically, and emotionally ready to compete. I've traveled with athletes who routinely stay at the same hotel, eat dinner at the same restaurant, eat the same breakfast, and use the same shower cubicle in the locker room at the particular tournament venue. These world-class athletes are creatures of habit and can be very superstitious.

Athletes: pre-competition routines ensure total preparation and optimum readiness for peak performance. Leading up to competition, following a routine helps eliminate distractions, manage nerves and anxiety, and focus the mind. Routines can create familiarity in unfamiliar places and they can create calm in pressure-filled situations.

American track and field athlete and Olympic gold medalist, Tianna Bartoletta, follows a pre-race routine that includes: getting to the venue two hours early to get a feel for the atmosphere, wearing headphones to listen to music as she warms up and stretches, and finding a quiet place to visualize and focus.

American swimmer and Olympic gold medalist, Michael Phelps, has followed the same pre-race routine since he was 11 years of age. He starts with 30 minutes of stretching and then gets in the pool for a 45 minute swim warm up of varying distances, drills, and speeds. He then changes from his warm up gear into his racing gear. He listens to music (hip hop, rap, or techno) for about 20 minutes to help him get focused for the upcoming race. In the final moments before the race, he stands behind his starting block for four minutes. When they announce his name, he steps onto and then back off of the starting block. He then swings his arms 3 times and steps back onto the block to get into his starting position.

Developing an effective pre-competition routine (*prepareadiness*) is a process. Over time you will fine-tune the routine into what works best for you. What works for a friend or a practice partner may work for them, but may not be what works for you. Develop your own, keep it simple, and follow it consistently.

* * *

*Champion minded athletes are creatures of habit.*

# Visualization

*Visualizing performance is reassuring and empowering for athletes.*

Visualization is an important part of preparation. It provides an internal and an external perspective on performance. Using visualization, or imagery, means seeing yourself from the inside looking out, as if you were actually performing your sport; or seeing yourself from the outside as though watching yourself perform. Good imagery is more than just the visual perspective. It includes the multi-sensory experience: the sights, sounds, smells, physical sensations, mental processes, and the emotional routines. Champion minded athletes imagine their success. Before it happens in reality, they see it happening in the mind. Visualization should be part of the daily routine and the competition routine.

Canadian bobsledder Lyndon Rush, said, "Before the Winter Olympics in Sochi, I drove the course hundreds of times in my mind. I've tried to keep the track in my mind throughout the year, " he said. "I'll be in the shower or brushing my teeth. It just takes a minute, so I do the whole thing, or sometimes just the corners that are more technical. You try to keep it fresh in your head, so when you do get there, you are not just starting at square one. It's amazing how much you can do in your mind."

Athletes: when you first start performing in your mind, your brain creates a neural pattern, one that your muscles will follow with practice and repetition. Commit three minutes per day to visualization, imagining yourself performing in specific venues for specific events and achieving your goals. Doing so will dramatically increase your chances for achieving in reality that which you have rehearsed in your mind.

Some years back, I worked with a world number 1 squash player. She always insisted on going to see the courts prior to competing in the tournament. She liked to have a clear image of the arena, the smells, they temperature, etc. She would then go to her room and visualize herself performing in that environment - seeing in her mind what she wanted to happen in reality. Similarly, after a training session in Copenhagen, three time Olympian in Badminton, Scott Evans, told me he would often use visualization as part of his preparation. He said: "I like to visualize the small details. Even things such as the eating facilities, where I'd be warming up, the court, etc. so that nothing would come to me as a surprise on match day."

* * *

*See it. Believe it. Work for it. Achieve it!*

*Using visualization can be a very powerful tool for athletes. Before it happens in reality, it must first happen in the mind.*

*"I was taught at a very young age to visualize. It was how I wanted it to go, how I didn't want it to go, and how it could go."*

- Michael Phelps

# Embrace the Butterflies

*Expect and embrace the nerves.*

As a five-time world championship competitor in the sport of Duathlon (running & cycling), I know what it is like to stand on a world championship start line. I also know what it feels like to have my stomach turning inside out and upside down! In fact, I almost missed the start of the 2002 World Championship race in Atlanta due to taking a last minute toilet stop!

Ask any athlete competing at the top, and they will tell you that they get nervous. Even those who have many years experience and who've won multiple world titles or Olympic medals, still get nervous every time they step up to the competition line!

Every athlete deals with nerves. Nerves are a sign that you care about what you are doing. If you are not nervous before competition, there's a problem. Feeling nervous is not a bad thing - it's fuel for your performance. It's evidence you are fired up and ready for action! Near the end of my competitive career, I was asked when I would know that it was time to walk away. I answered that when I no longer felt the butterflies, I would know it was over. Nerves showed me that what I was doing mattered!

Athletes - don't fight the nerves, use them for good! They indicate you are excited and ready to perform - that what you are doing is meaningful and important to you. Also, don't forget your opponents are going through the exact same thing!

Find that perfect *prepareadiness* routine (the systematic actions you take an hour before going out to compete). Having a familiar routine before going out to compete helps keep you focused and more relaxed. Of course you'll still feel some butterflies, but you'll be better equipped to handle them!

* * *

*Having nerves is a sign that what you are doing is meaningful and important to you.*
*Embrace them!*

# Mantras

*Champion minded athletes use mantras or buzzwords to stay focused.*

A mantra is a thought behind speech or action; a word or catchphrase repeated to aid concentration and focus. Champion minded athletes use mantras to encourage themselves and to help them stay focused on the task at hand. There won't always be a teammate, a coach, or a crowd to cheer you on - you've got to cheer for yourself.

To help let go of the last play and to focus their mind on the present after a missed shot, catch, kick, swing or putt, I advise players to say "forget and focus." Mantras serve as pre-competition concentration rituals, in-competition responses to help focus, calm, encourage, and celebrate. They also serve as post-competition rituals for mental and emotional recovery. Athletes must develop and train with these mantras. They are not reserved for competition.

When I competed in 7 marathons and half marathons in 7 weeks, I struggled around the 33 kilometer mark in my final race. I was dealing with some heat and hydration issues on that day. I said to myself, *"Every step I take is one step closer."* This simple one line mantra helped me get through the last few kilometers and to complete the final race.

During the 2016 Olympics Games in Rio, gymnast and gold medal winner Laurie Hernandez was seen whispering to herself, *"I got this"* before going on to help clinch the gold medal for team USA. Champion minded athletes choose mantras that are performance-based rather than outcome-based and therefore do not include words referring to outcomes such as *"win"* or *"lose."* Using outcome-based words increases anxiety and stress. Simple reminders are great: *focus, breathe, fight, relax,* and *let's go.* Affirmative statements are also beneficial: *I'm ready, I can do this,* and *I have what it takes.*

\* \* \*

## *"I got this!"*

- Laurie Hernandez, Olympic Gold Medalist in Gymnastics

# Competing Against a Friend

*Your opponents should be faceless.*

If you haven't already, there will come a time when you have to compete against a friend. It's not easy. I encountered this challenge throughout my junior career and up to the world championship level. I shared a hotel room with one of my fiercest rivals on our national team. We were friends and teammates, but when it came time to compete, we put on our game faces. Emotional toughness is related to, but separate from, mental toughness.

While mental and emotional toughness require routines and discipline, mental toughness is more analytical as it relates to decision making during competition, strategy, game-planning, implementing patterns of play, identifying strengths and weaknesses in opponents, analyzing whether to stick to the original plan or change the course of action, etc. Emotional toughness deals with the athlete's ability to handle anxiety, anger, fear, frustration, and panic. Emotional toughness is even more exposed when faced with adversity. The ability to close it out - to not choke, to overcome obstacles, to be resilient - is emotional toughness.

Grand Slam champion and former tennis world #1 Kim Clijsters was a master of emotional toughness. She was friendly and congenial off the court, but a fierce competitor on the court. She had an emotional toughness that allowed her to set all else aside from the task at hand - winning. Your opponent should be faceless. You are competing against an opponent, not a friend or an enemy. Assigning opponents to categories increases anxiety and creates stumbling blocks emotionally and mentally. Focus on the process and just play.

## 5 Tips for Emotional Toughness when competing:

1. Always show respect to your opponent, friend or not.

2. When you enter the competitive arena it's about competing, not friendship.

3. Approach each match with the same routines - keep the opponent faceless.

4. Keep your emotions in check by focusing on the game plan and task at hand.

5. Focus on controlling what you can control.

* * *

*Focus on the process and just compete.*

*Attitude is a choice.*
*Body Language is a choice.*
*Work Ethic is a choice.*
*Being coachable is a choice.*

# Simple Thinking Is Smart Thinking

*Champion minded athletes are able to simplify under pressure.*

C larity and simplicity are essential to managing pressure-filled competitive situations. The elite athletes of every sport develop personal routines and rituals to help them stay calm and focused during competition. When asked about fellow professional golfer Jordan Speith, seasoned player Brad Faxon said, "A lot of guys are looking for information to make things more complicated, but Jordan is always looking to make things simpler." Champion minded athletes process information in clear and simple terms, which leads to calm and composed performance.

A highly acclaimed Squash coach I was speaking to recently shares the same belief. He said, "As a player, when you are under pressure, always try to keep it simple. Don't overthink or plan too many things, just keep it simple."

Steve Hansen, coach of the winningest team in world sports, the All Blacks rugby team, also agrees, saying, "Our job is to make the complex simple. The simpler you can make it for somebody, the easier it is to do."

Remember the goal is not to make it complex, but to make it simple.

\* \* \*

*Always keep it simple under pressure.*

*The mind is everything. It can make you fail or win. If you're not mentally focused and in-control of your emotions, you'll fail.*

# Know What You Can Control

*Champion minded athletes focus on what they can control.*

The champion minded are able to do this one thing better than the rest - control the controllables. They don't waste energy on what they can't control.

By focusing on what you can control - your routines and habits, your effort, your discipline, your attitude, your self-talk, your coachable-ness, your behavior, your focus - you free yourself of stress, fear, and anxiety and you clear the path to realizing your potential.

Athletes who focus on what they cannot control - facility conditions, weather, the opponent, referees/officials, spectators, teammates, coaches, playing time, fans, results, others expectations/opinions - are more prone to be nervous, anxious, tense, fearful, and worried, which leads to poor performance.

As an athlete, it's so important to be aware of what you can control and what you cannot control. When uncontrollables start to lure you into negative thinking, recognize it, take a breath, and shift your focus back to what you can control in the present moment.

\* \* \*

*The average are easily distracted. The champion minded are locked in and focused.*

# How To Eat An Elephant

*"A journey of a thousand miles begins with a single step." - Confucius*

My father used to say, "How do you eat an elephant? Piece by piece." This is one of my favorite go-to phrases when facing an overwhelmingly large task. He was reminding me to take it one step at a time and to focus on the task at hand. Panic creeps in when we look beyond the task at hand and the enormity of the task ahead feels overwhelming. This shift in focus from the task at hand to the task ahead creates openings for the mind to wander and to create scenarios that haven't happened yet and which may never happen. Focusing on these hypothetical scenarios can sometimes make them become self-fulfilling prophesies.

Athletes: when you are feeling overwhelmed and panic starts to creep in, think of the elephant eating theory. If you're in the middle of a competition and you feel a flood of thoughts about the end result, return to the present moment and to the process. After claiming his 18th career Grand Slam title at the 2017 Australian Open, Roger Federer, said,

> It can sometimes be easy to think ahead when you are in a match, but what's important is you take it point by point and look no further. You play the ball, you don't play the opponent. You need to be free in your head, be free in your shots, and just go for it. The

*brave will be rewarded, you just need to stay
in the process and believe in it.*

Champion minded athletes take it one step at a time, not getting ahead of themselves. They stay focused in the moment and they trust the process. The next time you feel overwhelmed by the enormity of a task, just think about the elephant eating theory and take it piece by piece!

* * *

*"Faith is taking the first step even when you can't see
the whole staircase."*

- Martin Luther King, Jr.

# SECTION 6:

# *During Competition*

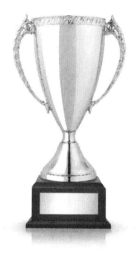

# Be Process Driven

*Champion minded athletes stay in the moment.*

After winning the 2014 British Open, world number one golfer Rory McIlroy spoke about his mindset and his approach going into the final round play. He mentioned the use of one simple word he kept repeating to himself: *process*. Each time he stepped up to play the next ball, he would remind himself to *just focus on the process*.

All too often, I see athletes overthink situations, making them more difficult and more complicated than necessary. Tennis legend, Arthur Ashe said famously, "There is a syndrome in sports called 'paralysis by analysis.'"

Overthinking often leads to over-trying, and it's the overthinking that fails you in the end.

A champion minded athlete stays in the present, and all that matters is what they are doing in that moment.

Stay in the present moment. Don't let your mind drift forwards or backwards. Use positive and helpful self-talk to help keep you engaged and focused. And just like Rory McIlroy did in that final round, keep it simple and stay process minded.

\* \* \*

*When you focus on the process,*
*the results take care of themselves.*

# Fear vs Fearless and Free

*The champion minded
aim to play freely and fearlessly.*

Before game five of the 2017 NBA championships, Golden State Warriors player, Kevin Durant, said in a pre-match interview that his goal was to play "free." He wanted to enjoy the moment and to just play his game. Durant mentioned that he hadn't been feeling that way all throughout the finals. Fast forward to the end of game five. Durant played his best game and won the finals MVP. He attributed the win to what he called, "playing fearless and playing free."

Playing with fear stems from being focused on the wrong things. It's about being fixated on the outcome and the result. It involves over-thinking. It's marked by self-doubt and a lack of confidence in personal ability and preparation. Playing with fear indicates a fixed mindset - being scared to make a mistake and afraid of losing. It's about trying to be perfect. It's this kind of thinking that cripples you physically and mentally.

Playing freely is about letting go and believing in yourself and your game. It's about focusing on the process, not the result. It's about trusting the work and the preparation you've put in. It's about enjoying the very act of competing and about challenging yourself. It's more about the doing and not the thinking. It's about putting in the continuous effort and then just letting it happen. Playing freely is about having a growth mindset, not being afraid to make mistakes, and aiming for progress, not perfection.

The champion minded always aim to play freely and fearlessly.

\* \* \*

*"Playing free" is about enjoying the very act of competing and challenging yourself.*

# Forget & (Re) Focus

*Champion minded athletes*
*are able to let go of mistakes and move on.*

Much time is spent on perfecting flawless technical skills. It is a necessity to develop fundamental techniques and tactics, however, too little time is spent on the skill of letting go and moving on from the last play, point, stroke, or game. During Tiger Woods' relentless domination during the early 2000's, his most important mental tool was the ability to let go of the last shot. He understood that his mental and emotional response was vitally important to the next play!  What you're thinking, what you're focusing on, how you're reacting to the previous play mentally and emotionally, is absolutely critical to the outcome.

Use my 'FF' mantra - "Forget" the last play and "Focus" on the next. The quicker you can do this, the better. I even have some athletes write it on their hand so they can see it during competition.

Champion minded athletes devote competition time to everything regarding play - the physical, the technical, the tactical skills at work. In order to stay fully present during actual play, champion minded athletes devote the time between plays to mental and emotional routines aimed at letting go of previous plays and preparing for next plays.  Mental awareness and emotional control massively impact the final outcome. The opponent may be bigger, stronger, faster, and more experienced, but if you have better control of your mind and your emotions, you will have the advantage.

M

* * *

*There's no point in dwelling on the last play. You can't bring it back. It's gone, move on!*

# Handling the Big Moments

*Champion minded athletes
treat all moments as Big Moments.*

Tom Rinaldi interviewed Jordan Spieth after his 2015 Master's win. He asked the young golfer how he handled those putts in the pressure moments. Spieth answered, "They are all big moments and putts, from the time I tee off, to the last ball. I see every shot I hit as equally important."

I asked head of performance at Manchester United Football Club, Tony Strudwick, how the players he worked with at one of the largest clubs in the world, handled the pressure moments, Tony said,

> *The champion players have an ability to win the moments that really matter. Right thing, right time, every time. However, this can only be achieved through a lifelong pursuit of mastery and excellence in their chosen sport. In other words, they prepare for these moments long before they happen. The champion performers are also able to control their emotions better.*

This is a great way of perceiving things. Like Tony said, you need to be prepared for it. If you highlight the bigger moments or points while competing, you only create anxiety and impose pressure upon yourself. The best way to handle these moments is to treat them the same. The champion minded see all competitive moments the same - they all count.

\* \* \*

*Be so involved in the process, that you even forget about the score!*

*Champion minded athletes stay in the moment and focus on the process. They don't get ahead of themselves.*

# Pressure is a Privilege

*Champion minded athletes
see pressure as an opportunity.*

T he year was 1981. In Johannesburg, South Africa, my parents took me to watch my first ever tennis match, featuring Billie Jean King. Billie Jean King is an American former World No. 1 professional tennis player. She won 39 Grand Slam titles, including 12 singles, 16 women's doubles, and 11 mixed doubles titles. King won the singles title at the inaugural WTA Tour Championships. Billie Jean King knows how to handle pressure. I recently read her book, *Pressure is a Privilege*, and found her perspective on pressure to be a great example for all athletes.

From recreational players to professional athletes, pressure is present for all ages and levels. Often, people view pressure as a burden. After reading Billie Jean King's book, I adopted a better perspective. Athletes: if you are experiencing pressure, it's because of your expectation to perform (either what you expect of yourself or what others expect of you). Expectation of performance means there is an anticipation of outcome. Outcomes are out of your control; however, you are in control of the effort you give. View expectations as a vote of confidence that you can perform and achieve a desired outcome. Use pressure to fuel your effort, but first eliminate expectations about outcome.

Avoiding pressure leads to underperformance and unrealized dreams. Athletes: if you are unwilling to test your own limits, you'll never reach your potential. It is performance under pressure that leads to great accomplishment. Champion minded athletes embrace pressure and nerves and they use them to their advantage. They use positive rituals and self-talk to combat the pressure and to use it for their gain. You can convince yourself that you are at your best when under pressure. Pressure can be the adrenalin for your success.

* * *

*"Pressure is a privilege,*
*an opportunity to achieve greatness."*

- Billie Jean King

# Don't Listen to Yourself, Talk to Yourself!

## *Positive self-talk is an essential skill.*

During competition, and especially when dealing with fatigue, it's more important to talk to yourself than to listen to yourself. When pressured, stressed or tired, there might be a voice in your head complaining about the temperature, body aches, or the effort it will take to continue. Doubt creeps in, uncertainty hovers, the desire to just be *done* can feel overwhelming! But these are self-defeating thoughts. Do not listen to them. By talking to yourself, you have the ability to drown out the inner voices of doubt.

Champion minded athletes have trained themselves to be their own biggest motivators and supporters. They are their own positive self-coach constantly talking into their ear, telling them they can do it!

When they talk to themselves, these champion minded athletes know what to say. They understand that developing this kind of mindset takes practice. They work on developing a positive language and dialogue with themselves constantly.

Building a great mindset is not a sometimes thing. It is an all-the-time thing. Much like how individuals revert to their worst habits under pressure, so too, does the quality of thoughts and self-talk. If you are always berating yourself for mistakes and errors during practice, you will do that during competition also. No matter how good your game skills are, a negative mindset will always hinder your progress.

Develop a powerful self-talk, one that builds you up, not one that breaks you down. Doing so takes time, effort, and practice, but it's of vital importance. The champion minded are serial self-talkers. They are their own positive self-coaches!

\* \* \*

*In challenging times, champion minded athletes have trained themselves to be their own biggest motivators.*

# Go To Your Notes

*We all need reminders
to help us get back on track and refocus.*

It's impossible to remember everything. Thats why I find it so important to write things down. As speakers keep note cards or as actors have cue cards, so too should athletes have notes. In a pressure situation, it's easy to lose track and become overwhelmed by the occasion. Along the way, we all need reminders in order to stay focused and on the right track, especially in the pressure-filled environment of competition. While writing my first book, *7 Keys to Being a Great Coach,* I spent lots of time observing some of the world's best athletes and coaches. Most of these top performers would refer to their notes as a way to stay focused on the game plan and remember to go back to the basics and fundamentals, especially in pressure-filled moments. I like to call these reminders "go-to notes."

Some great examples include Grand Slam champions such as Serena Williams and Andy Murray, who can be often seen reading hand-written notes on change-overs during a match. Legendary quarterbacks Peyton Manning and Tom Brady also go to their notes during the game. NBA basketball star, Kyle Korver, even has a checklist, including 21 pointers to help remind him of his shooting technique. Many notes include an athlete's technical or tactical tips. They also include some motivational and mindset messages.

If the very best in the world need reminders, then all of us do. With that in mind, it's good to have a note book or a card with some key fundamentals written down to help remind you. Just like the champion minded performers mentioned in this chapter, we all need reminders to stay focused and on track - especially in stressful situations.

* * *

*The champion minded*
*keep notes and reminders to help them succeed.*

# Relentless

*Champion minded athletes are relentless in their pursuit of greatness.*

Back in 2013, I went to go watch Alison Waters, a former squash player I had the privilege to help a few times while residing in Amsterdam, compete. At one point, the likable Alison reached number 3 in the world rankings. At the British National Squash Championships in Manchester, England I watched a few of her matches. That week, Alison played exceptionally well and took home the national title. After congratulating her on claiming her maiden British title, I inquired about her mindset on the court that week. I was fascinated by her intensity and focus. In addition to believing in herself, she repeatedly told herself, *"Be relentless."* During all of her 5 matches that week, Alison had focused on that one powerful mantra - *be relentless.*

To be relentless is to be unyielding - to persist. Champion minded athletes never let up during competition. They don't allow their opponents to breathe. They keep their foot on the pedal until the competition is done. They are aware of how quickly momentum can shift, and they do not falter. Champion minded athletes press on toward their goal without giving up or giving in. They don't give their opponents an inch. Like Alison was that week in Manchester, they are relentless!

\* \* \*

*The champion minded are relentless when they compete. They don't give their opponents an inch.*

# Your Negativity Gives Your Opponent Hope

*The champion minded protect their image.*

**Athletes - be aware that the opposition is energized and motivated by your:**

1. Negativity
2. Poor Body Language
3. Doubtfulness
4. Poor Preparation
5. Bad Attitude
6. Lack of Effort
7. Poor Self-Talk
8. Poor Discipline
9. Lack of Work Ethic
10. Lack of Focus

\* \* \*

*Let go of behaviors and beliefs that
no longer serve you well.*

# Grit

*Have the endurance, perseverance,
and passion to stay committed.*

In my experience working with many elite athletes, I've observed that the physical and technical differences among top athletes are very small. The top athletes are all physically fit, they have trained athletic skills, they have developed sport-specific skills, and they are good competitors. Otherwise, they wouldn't be at the top. If you went to a golf driving range or to tennis practice courts to watch the top 100 players in the world practice, you probably wouldn't be able to tell the difference between a player ranked 10 or 100 - they all have sound fundamental technique and are all physically fit.

I'm often asked what separates the good from the great athletes. The short answer is grit. In her TED talk, "Grit: The Power of Passion and Perseverance" Angela Lee Duckworth defines grit as, "self-discipline, combined with a passionate commitment to a task and a burning desire to see it through." As a coach, I've never come across an athlete who has reached an elite level without overcoming obstacles. The struggle to overcome difficulty builds grit. Grit isn't inherent, but it can be developed. Just as physical, mental, and emotional skills can be trained and developed, so too can grit grow and evolve. Developing grit is a long process. It does not happen in one training session. All along the journey, as challenges arise, athletes develop grit.

Athletes - when challenges and difficulties occur, don't shy away from them. Instead, face them head on and persist! Remember, it takes courage to develop grit. Champion minded athletes understand that there are valuable lessons in defeat, and perseverance is essential for success. Attitude is a choice. When faced with difficulty, choose to be resilient. Choose grit.

* * *

*Champion minded athletes view struggle and obstacles as a great way to develop grit.*

*A champion minded athlete views pressure, fatigue, and struggle as ways to build greater resilience and grit. They see opportunity in difficulty.*

# Resilience

*Champion minded athletes embrace the struggle now for victory later.*

Before we address resilience in sport, let's address resilience in life. The American Psychological Association defines resilience as:

> *...the process of adapting well in the face of adversity, trauma, tragedy, threats, or even significant sources of stress - such as family and relationship problems, serious health problems, or workplace and financial stressors.*

It means bouncing back from difficult experiences.

When soccer star Lionel Messi turned 11, his life changed. He was diagnosed with growth hormone deficiency. A local team was interested in him and his skills, however they could not afford to cover the costs of the treatments his condition required: $900 a month, which is a fortune in this part of Argentina. This setback created something magnificent. Rather than discourage him, Messi let it motivate him and he developed a powerful mindset. The "poor me" attitude and excuses or complaints never appeared. Instead, he focused on becoming unbeatable in the game he loved and on growing as a person. Today, he is an ambassador for UNICEF and he has created his own charitable foundation.

I asked Wasps and England rugby fly-half, Danny Cipriani, what being champion minded meant to him. Danny said, "Resilience. The ability to keep coming back after being knocked down. Coming back stronger from defeats. It's the mental strength and resilience that sets the true champions apart, I believe."

My good friend, Michael Joyce, coach to world number one players, Maria Sharapova and Victoria Azarenka, told me over lunch, that the best athletes all had an ability to bounce back quicker from disappointments. They were incredibly resilient and they always refused to give in.

6-time Olympian and 4-time gold medalist in Ice Hockey, Hayley Wickenheiser, said that all of the champion minded athletes she'd played and worked with had been incredibly resilient. They all had the ability to adapt to any circumstance and to perform on demand. No matter what the circumstances, they could find ways to win.

\* \* \*

*"It's the mental strength and resilience that sets the true champions apart."*

- Danny Cipriani

# Champions Play Hard Until the Final Whistle

### *Champion minded athletes never let up or give in.*

A refusal to surrender separates the good and the great athletes. Champion minded athletes fight to the bitter end. They never let up. Have you ever watched champions such as tennis great Serena Williams, squash star Mohamed El Shorbagy, or Formula One race car driver Lewis Hamilton seem to find a way to win in what seems like a hopeless situation? How are they able to seize victory from the clutches of defeat? Champion minded athletes know how difficult it can be to close out a match, race, bout, or game, and they fight even harder in those pivotal and desperate moments. Their refusal to yield gains them wins. When victory is in your sight, have you ever experienced the feeling of hoping and wishing for your opponent to give up and to give you the win? These are dangerous thoughts. Champion minded athletes are aware of this temptation, but they stay process driven.

When faced with what seems to be certain defeat, mentally weak athletes quit trying. They lose hope, they abandon the will to fight, and they give up before the final buzzer or final point. In their minds, it's over before it's actually over. Champion minded athletes know how quickly momentum can shift in competition and they never concede a loss. To force their opponents to *earn* victory, champion minded athletes battle relentlessly. They never quit.

Sir Alex Ferguson is a former Scottish football manager and player who managed Manchester United from 1986 to 2013. Many players, managers, and analysts regard him as the greatest and most successful manager of all time. During his 26 years with Manchester United, he won 38 trophies, including 13 Premier League titles, 5 FA Cups, and 2 UEFA Champions League titles. To describe his teams' penchant for winning in the last few minutes of a game, commentators coined the phrase "Fergie time." He coached his teams to be aware of the opponents' tendencies to let up when nearing the end of play and of their habit to think the match is over before time expires. He taught them to capitalize on these opportunities and to attack in those final moments. That is a great lesson for any athlete or team!

* * *

*"I've never lost a game, I just ran out of time."*

- Michael Jordan

# SECTION 7:

# *After Competition*

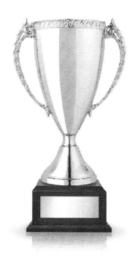

.

# Celebrate Small Successes

*"Nothing succeeds like success"*
*Justin Timberlake (feat. Jay Z) "Suit & Tie"*

W hat do you think most retired athletes regret the most from their careers? They wish they had taken more time to enjoy the journey and to celebrate small successes along the way. In pursuit of greater achievements and bigger accomplishments, they would reach a small goal and just move on to the next goal without stopping.

I was the same. When competing on the international triathlon circuit, I would often have a great result but would fail to celebrate it - it was just never good enough! I also wish I had realized, before my career ended, that success entails a certain state of mind - working hard, but also enjoying the rewards brought on by the work done.

Celebrating small successes builds confidence, which strengthens mental toughness. Celebrating small success does not mean being content or complacent. Rather, it accelerates the momentum towards accomplishing the next goal. Celebration is relative - small successes should be recognized with small rewards, bigger wins should be celebrated with bigger rewards. Implement a reward system for yourself that reflects the achievement.

Success breeds success. Stop focusing on what's going wrong and focus on what's going well. Celebrate the daily wins in your routines. In order to stay motivated throughout the process, set attainable short-term goals within the larger context of bigger long-term goals. It's a long journey to reach the final destination. Take time to celebrate the small successes along the way and you'll enjoy the journey!

## 3 Reasons to Celebrate Small Successes:

1. Celebrating small successes builds momentum, confidence, and self-belief.

2. Celebrating small successes motivates you to work towards the next goal.

3. Celebrating small successes trains you to think and act like a champion.

* * *

*Celebrating the small successes builds momentum, confidence and self-belief.*

# Champions Hate Losing More Than They Love Winning

*The fear of losing can sometimes be a powerful motivator.*

Champion minded athletes hate to lose more than they love to win. When sports psychologist Brooke MacNamara was asked to comment on the common traits of the most decorated Olympians, she listed competitiveness and the will to win as major factors. She explained further, "Some people hate to lose more than they love to win. Either way it's a powerful motivator." Over the last 20 years, every athlete I have worked with has shared this trait. If you don't hate losing, you probably aren't willing to do the things necessary to avoid it. Jimmy Conners, the tennis great once said, "I hate to lose more than I love to win."

Champion minded athletes hate losing. How they respond to losing is another factor that distinguishes the good from the great. There is suffering, anger, frustration, disappointment, regret, and sadness attached to defeat. Champion minded athletes learn and grow from it.

How an athlete responds to defeat - immediately, and in the days following - matters. In the immediate moments of defeat, stay classy, be respectful, and congratulate your opponent no matter what. Defeat hurts - you should feel pain. Defeat is also a test of character. How an athlete bounces back from a loss is important.

The champion minded are able to move on quickly and to learn from their losses.

\* \* \*

*"Above anything else, I hate to lose."*

\- Jackie Robinson

*Winning a championship is not as important as who you become on the journey to becoming a champion.*

# How Sweet It Is

*Hard work beats talent*
*when talent doesn't work hard.*

When an athlete realizes that consistent effort, a positive attitude, and superior work ethic can defeat a more talented player, an epiphany may occur.

Knowing the opponent may be more skilled and experienced than you can be daunting. Knowing you have the the edge because of your diligence, discipline, and grit can empower you. The feeling of all those extra hours of work you've put in, the extra sweat, the tears - are now paying off.

\* \* \*

*"There may be people who have more talent than you,*
*but there's no excuse for anyone to work harder than*
*you do – and I believe that."*

- Derek Jeter

# Doubt

## *Doubt is a thief!*

Doubt begins with negative and unproductive thoughts that lead to a breakdown of confidence. Doubt halts your momentum. Self-doubt interferes with your performance in two ways. First, your focus shifts from external real-time performance to internal worry about what has already happened and what the future outcome will be. As a result, you lose awareness of important performance-relevant cues. Your concentration shifts from the only thing within your control - the present moment - to things beyond your control, such as what has already happened and what has yet to happen. Second, self-doubt interferes with your ability to perform due to direct physiological reactions - difficulty breathing, muscle tension, nervousness, increase in heart rate, etc.

Overcoming doubt starts with positive self-talk. Keep reminding yourself that you have what it takes to succeed. Remind yourself of all the work you have done to get ready for this moment. Preparation is the foundation of confidence and a tool that can help you conquer doubt.

When I asked English International cricket player, Sam Billings, about the subject he replied, "I think every athlete goes through periods of doubt in their career. It's only human. You need to trust the work and preparation you've put in and stop doubting it. It's also important to keep a perspective on things and have fun. It's something you learn over time."

Facebook founder, Mark Zuckerberg, admitted he too was plagued by self-doubt. In his 2017 Harvard commencement speech, Zuckerberg said that his solution to beating it was to find a higher purpose and keep believing in his long-term vision.

In times of self-doubt, a good strategy is to surround yourself with people who believe in you and who remind you of your good preparation and capabilities. Visualize your past successes, and use those visions as inspiration and motivation. Use your energy to stay positive in the present moment and to conquer self-doubt. Doubt is nothing more than a little voice in your head that needs to be silenced. Don't let it prevent you from doing great things!

\* \* \*

*"Stay true to your long-term purpose and work your hardest until you achieve it."*

- Mark Zuckerberg

*When you start doubting yourself,
remember how far you've come -
all the battles you've won and all the
fears you've overcome.*

# What is Defeat?

*Champion minded athletes find victory even in defeat.*

Champion minded athletes compete to win. They don't give up and they don't give in. Part of this determination is the ability to find victory even in defeat. When champion minded athletes lose, they are able to move on quickly from the pain and disappointment of losing and to recognize the lessons to be learned and see the opportunities for growth. Learning from mistakes is part of mastery.

In life and in sport, there will be struggle. There will be hard times. Champion minded athletes learn from losses and return to training, re-dedicated to improving. They are able to analyze losses and to use the information to make adjustments that will lead to better future performance. Defeat in attitude and actions, defines lesser minded athletes. Their negative response to defeat becomes their greatest obstacle to success. This is true in life and in sport.

Growth stems from struggle. If you only do what you are already good at doing, you'll never grow beyond that point. It takes courage to put yourself out there - to try for something more than what you have already accomplished. Trying and failing is an opportunity to learn and to improve.

* * *

*"What is defeat? Nothing but education, nothing but the first step to getting better."*

- Vince Lombardi

*After a defeat, average players look at the umpires, conditions, coaches, or teammates to place blame while champion minded athletes look at themselves and assess what they could have done better or differently.*

# How to Best Handle Defeat

*Defeat reveals your character.*

A few years ago I was invited to watch a squash tournament at Harvard University in Boston. There was a young player who had been tipped for great things, and I wanted to see him in action. The match was a tough and at times nasty affair, and neither player wanted to give the other an inch. What I remember most about the match was the following: the player I went to watch lost the match and stormed off the court without shaking his opponent's hand. Even though he was a great player, his behavior in defeat was not appropriate.

Most of us who have lost a close, hard-fought match know disappointment - sometimes it really hurts. One of the most accurate judges of a person's character is how he or she handles defeat. Champion minded athletes hate to lose, but they are always graceful in defeat. When champion minded teams or athletes lose, they do so with dignity, respect, and class.

Athletes - how you respond to defeat reveals your true character. Yes, losing hurts. But, as painful as defeat can be, you must always find it within yourself to sincerely congratulate your opponent. Tennis great Rafael Nadal is a great role model. I watched him lose an epic match at the U. S. Open and though devastated, he warmly congratulated his opponent with a handshake and an embrace. And then, upon leaving the court, he took time to sign autographs for fans - a true class act!

Show respect to whomever has defeated you. Shake hands with your opponent, and congratulate him or her on a job well done. This is how you earn respect.

The fact is, you can't win them all. The greats of the game hate to lose, but they also know it is inevitable. So, they learn to move on and to take the lessons as they come. Even in defeat, they display gratitude to those who help and support them. They also don't make excuses for why they lost. Always be of good character and your reputation will take care of itself.

* * *

*When champion minded teams or athletes lose, they do so with dignity, respect, and class.*

*No matter how strong or weak your opposition may be, prepare, respect and treat them all the same.*

# Difference Between Failing & Being a Failure

*No one grows in comfort.*

When it comes to dealing with defeat or failure, there are two kinds of people. The first type are those who see failure as defeat, and then there are those who see the positives and learn from them.

Elon Musk, inventor, engineer, and CEO of SpaceX, said "Failure is an option. If things are not failing, you are not innovating enough." Recently, I read an article on the U.S. Army and their training methods. Lt. Col Ken Dilg of the US Army explains that we learn the most through our failures. When we push ourselves through the toughest times, we grow. If you ask a group of people what the toughest times in their lives were and at what times in their lives they grew and learned the most, there's a good chance those occasions will match up.

Every experience and trial provides us with lessons on how to get better and how to learn from mistakes or defeat. You have a choice. You can forget about the experience and sweep it under the carpet, or you can face up to it and plan for more success next time. How you deal with these experiences determines how far you can go.

No one grows in comfort. To strive for more we need to stretch ourselves. Sometimes that involves failing along the way. However, from failure and defeat we grow stronger. Having a growth mindset and embracing these challenges is what makes a champion minded athlete.

## Being a Failure (fixed mindset):

- ability is fixed and unchanging
- when tested, give up and quit
- avoid hard work and challenge

## Failing (growth mindset):

- there is always the possibility of improving
- a defeat is a temporary setback, part of the journey
- a loss is a motivating factor to work hard and try again

\* \* \*

*"Don't be afraid of failure. This is the way to succeed."*

- Lebron James

# A Champion Minded Approach To Failure

*Champion minded athletes
come back from failure more determined.*

**How a champion minded athlete approaches failure:**

**F** – First, identity what went wrong.

**A** – Always focus on the facts.

**I** – Improve from it.

**L** – Learn from it.

**U** – Understand it.

**R** – Renew the attitude.

**E** – Enter a new mindset ready to move on.

# Dealing with Disappointment

*Champion minded athletes
practice their responses to disappointment.*

How you respond to disappointment in life and in sport is directly linked to your attitude and mindset. Your responses need to be trained and practiced regularly. How do you move on in order to do better next time? Bouncing back from disappointment is not always easy!

## Here are 5 steps to help you move on:

1. Champion minded athletes allow themselves to feel the pain of disappointment, but then they let it go. Disappointment is natural. It shows that you care. When you are giving your best effort and you don't get the desired result, it is very difficult to forget about it immediately. Allow yourself some space for a natural emotional response. Give yourself time to decompress and to calm down. By feeling the disappointment, you can then release it and let it go. Experiencing disappointment only makes victory that much sweeter.

2. Rather than a stumbling block, champion minded athletes view disappointment as a stepping stone. If you don't release the feelings of disappointment, they will continue to weigh you down with more frustration and negativity. Instead of letting it fester and drag you farther away from your goal, use the disappointment as fuel to motivate you to move forward.

3. Champion minded athletes are aware that disappointment provides an opportunity to make changes and to adapt. They use the loss to learn how to handle difficult situations in the future. Initially, disappointments may set you back, but move forward and use them as valuable feedback.

4. Champion minded athletes reset quickly. They feel the disappointment and then release it. They use it as motivation to get one step closer to the goal. They are able to find a positive and to learn from difficult situations.

5. Champion minded athletes are process driven, not outcome driven. They understand that failure is a part of success. Disappointments are valuable experiences that help you come back stronger and more prepared for the next time you are pushed to your limits.

* * *

*Champion minded athletes see a setback as an opportunity for a great comeback.*

# Lessons from Losses

*You have never lost if you have learned.*

Michael Phelps is the most dominant swimmer ever to compete. How he handled defeat contributed to his success. After a loss in the 100m butterfly to Ian Crocker during the 2003 World Championships, Phelps taped a picture of Crocker onto his wall for daily motivation. In the next three Olympic Games (2004, 2008 and 2012), Phelps went on to win gold medals in the 100m butterfly.

During the 2012 Olympics, Phelps suffered a devastating loss in his signature event, the 200m butterfly. Over a nine-year span leading up to the London Olympic Games, when he was upset by South African Chad le Clos by .05 of a second, he had won 60 straight 200m butterfly events. Later, Phelps said, "I was so anti-watching that race, because I just didn't even want to bring up the memories." He did eventually watch and analyze the race, saying, "I noticed a lot that what I did in that race that I'm not going to do again. I think I'm a lot more prepared this time."

Another great example of learning from a tough loss comes from one of the world's best female golfers, Lexi Thompson. Playing in the 2017 LPGA Ladies ANA Inspiration tournament, a bizarre ruling prevented her from cruising to what looked like her second major title. A television viewer's email had alerted officials to a day-old rules violation, which penalized Thompson for a 1-inch ball placement error. The 4-shot penalty wiped out her 3-shot lead. Lexi eventually lost in the playoff, but her attitude during her post round interview was remarkable. Many young players could learn from her mindset. Lexi said, "Every day is a learning process." She then stopped to sign dozens of autographs after her heartbreak. "I wasn't expecting what happened today, but... it happens, and I'll learn from it and hopefully do better." Just three weeks later, Lexi won her next LPGA tour event at the Kingsmill Championship in Williamsburg, Virginia. A champion minded comeback!

Despite the pain of a defeat or misfortune, champion minded athletes, like Lexi and Michael, use these unfortunate experiences as learning opportunities and as motivation to improve their performances. Sometimes our losses teach us more about life than sports. Developing good sportsmanship (as Lexi showed), a positive attitude, self-discipline, teamwork, accountability, persistence, and resilience, builds character and prepares you for life's challenges.

* * *

*"Everyday is a learning process."*

\- Lexi Thompson

*We don't fail from our mistakes,*
*we fail from not learning from them.*

# Experiencing Setbacks

*Champions minded athletes*
*turn obstacles into stepping stones.*

In my 25 years of coaching and consulting, I've never met a successful athlete or individual who didn't experience setbacks and difficulties during their journey in sport or in life. The road to athletic greatness is not marked by perfection. Greatness comes from the ability to constantly overcome adversity and failure. Champion minded athletes turn obstacles into stepping stones.

Failure, disappointment, frustration, injury, and defeat become opportunities to grow stronger. To experience a setback is to experience a moment of possibility, a chance to develop grit and toughness. Champion minded athletes approach setbacks with a positive attitude for long-term growth and progress.

Every elite athlete I know has dealt with disappointments, hard losses, and injury. Response to setbacks is a major distinguishing factor between the good and the great in their respective sports. Champion minded athletes view setbacks as chances to learn, to improve, to re-focus, and to move forward stronger, wiser, and more resilient.

Former US Davis Cup tennis player, James Blake once said: "My greatest professional successes occurred after I had faced my most personal challenges. I used to think this was ironic. Now I realize that success flows directly from having cleared those hurdles."

When those tough challenges arise - and they will - the champion minded don't give up, don't make excuses, and don't place blame. They understand that failing is not the opposite of success, but rather, a part of it. They also know that how they handle the inevitable obstacles and setbacks determines their level of success.

\* \* \*

*Champion minded athletes*
*turn setbacks into even greater comebacks.*

# Regaining Confidence

*All great athletes
experience times of uncertainty and doubt.*

Professional athletes have reached the elite levels of their sport through hard work, dedication, and a relentless desire to be the best. They are meticulous in their efforts to get to the top and stay at the top. Training confidence is an essential part of the process. Belief can take your game to the next level.

1. *Let you faith be greater than your fear.* Fear is a powerful emotion, and when you succumb to fear, your performance suffers. The only way to stop making mistakes is to stop playing. Allow yourself to make mistakes, to learn from them, and never give up.

2. *Do what you do best.* Hit your favorite shot and enjoy the moment. Do it again. Feel comfort in the familiarity of a favorite pattern or play. Gain confidence through your strengths.

3. *Preparation is the foundation of confidence.* Tennis legend, Arthur Ashe said, "One important key to success is self-confidence. An important key to self-confidence is preparation."

4. *Get a boost from your support system.* It's hard to achieve success without a great support team. To have people cheering you on - family, friends, coaches, teammates - it helps tremendously to have people you can turn to for support and encouragement.

5. *Visualize past success.* Go to past victories - big and small - to remind you of past hard work that paid off. There is validation in past achievements which required great effort. Small

victories lead to bigger victories. Past success helps lead to future success.

When US Olympic swimmer and winner of five medals at the London Olympics, Alison Schmidt, was going through a confidence crisis at the U.S. Nationals in 2015, it was none other than Michael Phelps himself who advised her to watch some videos of her races from the London Olympics. He then advised her to visualize what she needed to do to get back to where she was.

* * *

*Self-confidence comes down to what you think, what you tell yourself, and what you believe about yourself.*

*"Confidence is everything. Sometimes you wake up and nothing goes well. But if you bring the right mindset and belief in what you've worked for, the edge comes back."*

- Grigor Dimitrov

# Dealing with Injury

*A time-out from the game can be an advantage.*

There are two guarantees in life: death and taxes. For athletes there are three: death, taxes and injury. Any world class athlete will tell you that there is a very fine line between being in peak condition and being injured.

Injuries are a part of an elite athlete's journey. Injury can be difficult to accept and should be treated as an obstacle to overcome. Injuries also present an opportunity to work on areas of training which can be improved while in a limited physical condition. Injury may pause competition and limit practice, but it does not have to prevent training altogether. Even when sidelined, champion minded athletes look for ways to improve.

Athletes: in the event of an injury, shift your focus to what you can do and shift away from what you cannot do. For example, if a lower limb is injured, you can still work your upper body and core. If there is an upper body injury, you may still be able to work on leg strength. As a coach, injuries reveal to me (and to the team) an athlete's drive, determination, and mental toughness. It starts with attitude, and attitude is your choice.

Even in a limited capacity, champion minded athletes choose to stay positive and to continue to work. The oldest comeback player ever on the women's professional tennis tour, Kimiko Date, age 47, said that when sidelined with injury, she felt more motivated to come back stronger than ever!

Champion minded athletes, like Kimiko, understand that the injury gives them time to focus on factors of their game they might otherwise not have trained. It's an opportunity to come back refreshed, stronger, and more determined!

We have also seen that time away from the game can change an athlete's perspective on life. In 2017, Wimbledon champion, Petra Kvitova, was forced to take time-out from the game after a house intruder attacked her. Petra mentioned that the time away had given her some new perspectives on life and changed her for the better. While recovering and rehabbing from an achilles injury, US Squash star, Amanda Sobhy said, "Life can be short and we need to take full advantage of every day, every minute, and every second we have."

Sometimes, in life, we need those hard knocks to make us more appreciative.

\* \* \*

*When injured, champion minded athletes focus on what they CAN DO.*

# 5 Things to Do When You're in a Slump

*Face challenges with courage and strength.*

During your career, it's inevitable that you'll experience performance slumps. All top athletes have gone through dips in performance. When this occurs, it's important not to panic.

The champion minded are always looking for the positives in adverse situations. They use setbacks to produce greater comebacks. When it comes to performance slumps, the difference between champion minded athletes and the rest is their ability to maintain an optimistic and a positive attitude. Slumps are like speed bumps. They slow you down for bit, but then it's time to put your foot on the gas.

## 5 Things to do When You're in a Slump:

1. **Less is more.** The most common response to a slump is to work harder and to practice more, but actually, this can be counterproductive. Give yourself some space, take a step back. I've witnessed players practicing less and getting better simply because they found a renewed enjoyment with less pressure to perform.

2. **Focus on your strengths and do what you enjoy.** Rekindle what you love about the game. Find what is fun, and bring your enjoyment of the game back. Remind yourself of when you were playing at your best - that was fun, right? Athletes: do what you love to do. Focus on the more fun exercises, drills, and games

you like to perform. Because your confidence stems from your strengths, practice your strengths more than your weaknesses.

3. **Surround yourself with good people.** When experiencing a slump, encouragement, assurance, and affirmation are so important. You need optimists around you. A slump is not the time for tough talk (unless of course it's needed due to laziness or a poor attitude). Surround yourself with people who will remind you that you have what it takes to succeed!

4. **Get your self-talk going.** Your self-talk is so important. Remember that what you say to yourself affects your confidence, which affects your performance. You can talk yourself into or out of almost anything. Stop feeling sorry for yourself. A slump is no time for self-pity. Speak, think and act like a champion.

5. **Stop over thinking it!** This is a big one. By over thinking things, you actually make them worse. Keep it simple, and keep your mind on the process. Stay in the moment, let go of past frustrations, and don't worry about the future result. Be patient and give it your best in the present time.

*Don't confuse mental toughness with working hard. Working hard is easy, but mental toughness is the amount of resilience and discipline present under adversity.*

# Ignore the Hype

### *Stay focused on the process.*

So often in the sports world we hear about young prodigies racing through the ranks. Over the past 25 years of my coaching career, I've witnessed some incredibly gifted young athletes succumb to the pressures and the expectations of others. In many cases, early success can be more of a curse than a blessing. Young athletes: don't be concerned if you're not the best player on your team. Remember, everyone develops at a different rate - physically, mentally, and emotionally. Instead, be concerned about getting better everyday. This is what a champion mindset is all about - constant self-improvement.

If you're the best player on the team or if you've had a great match, then resist the hype that comes with it. Don't let your ego be bigger than your drive to improve. Stay patient and focused on the process, the small successes, and the greater goal. Surround yourself with people who will insulate you from the outside noise and who will help you stay true to yourself. Trust the process and don't get ahead of yourself. Remember that the journey to athletic greatness is not a sprint, but a marathon. Excellence is not about a few good results, but rather, consistency over time.

Ignore what is said on social media. One week you can score the winning point and be hailed as a hero, and the next week you can miss the same shot and be the object of an online attack. Realize you are not defined by what you do, but rather, by who you are. Stay focused on your journey and aim to keep improving.

The champion minded athlete understands that doing their best today sets them up for success tomorrow. Expectations come with no guarantee. Stay champion minded and simply aim to be better than you were the day before.

* * *

*Remember that the journey to athletic greatness is a marathon not a sprint.*

*It's futile comparing your progress to others. Everybody has their own path. Stay focused on yours and trust the process.*

# Dealing with The Haters

*Champion minded athletes*
*rise above the critics, naysayers, and trolls.*

Haters are like crickets. They all make a lot of noise. You hear them, but you can't see them. When you walk past them, they're quiet.

Every time Basketball star Lebron James, or "King James" as he's known, plays away from home; the opposition's fans taunt and vilify him. Other athletes such as football star Ronaldo, and the most winning quarterback ever, Tom Brady, are also reviled regularly. Why is this? Because they are winners and feared. Champion athletes accept that there are many people who want to see them fail.

When I asked a former South African rugby player with whom I consulted in Johannesburg how he dealt with all the trolls and haters, he said, "I see them as a form of motivation. They actually inspire me to work even harder!"

Social media makes athletes, teams, and coaches accessible to fans and haters like never before. Fan is short for *fanatic,* and social media offers a platform for fanaticism. Fans are passionate. At times they go to far, becoming extreme in their social media attacks and rants. Foul language, racial slurs, and death threats are just some of the extreme, and extremely inappropriate opinions shared on social media. The world of fandom can get very ugly. At all levels though, athletes will deal with some sort of online criticism.

## How to Handle Haters:

1.  Don't engage. Just ignore it. This seems simple enough, but it is easier said than done. There is a natural tendency to want to respond to a challenge, to defend yourself, to prove or to justify your point. But why give validation to a stranger by engaging in an argument? Responding is not worth it.

2.  Block them. Use this great feature to stop someone from from posting attacks and abusive language. It eliminates the distraction, allowing athletes to place attention on positive messages instead of hateful rhetoric. Don't subject yourself to the toxic fanatics.

Haters are a fact of life and not everyone is going to be a fan of you. They hide behind computers and phone screens, and say things they would never have the courage to say in person. Haters are hoping to provoke a response. They are looking for a reaction. Don't give it to them. They do not deserve your attention, nor a response.

\* \* \*

*Work hard in silence. Let success be your noise.*

*The one thing you'll discover about a champion is that the more the haters and critics try knock them down, the stronger and better they keep coming back.*

# Some Good Advice from A World Champion

Four-time world long jump champion, Dwight Phillips, who earned a reputation as one of the sport's ultimate competitors, is Stanford University's track coach and a good friend of mine. 2004's Olympic champion, Dwight passes on three pieces of wisdom he learned during his stellar career.

## 1. Stay Disciplined.

The sport never came as naturally to me as to some of my colleagues, so I understood the importance of being disciplined. I was a late bloomer. I definitely saw the benefit of being fully disciplined from my junior year at college. From this year I paid more attention to my nutrition and my strength work in the weight room, and this year from the age of 17 to 18 it made a big difference. I went from an unknown with a long jump PB of 7.28m, to one of the best athletes in the world with a best of 8.18m. I was aware that there were kids better than me, so to be as good as them I paid attention to detail and I flourished. To deliver my dreams of appearing in the Sydney Olympics I knew I had to be razor sharp focused, start eating right and trust in my coach. All of that helped me make my first Olympic team in Sydney.

## 2. Never Stop Learning.

At the 2000 Olympics I competed purely off emotion and I had very little technical knowhow. So in an effort to be better, I started studying all the great jumpers from Bob Beamon to Ralph Boston and Mike Powell to Carl Lewis, and discovered there was an art to jumping. There were things they were doing consistently that I needed to integrate into my performance, if I wanted longevity in the sport. The U.S. had a great legacy in the long jump and I wanted to maintain that legacy, so I studied like I was a student at school and took the same approach to the long jump as I did completing my degree in broadcast communications. This to me made a huge difference and definitely contributed to my long-term success and longevity. I came up with different drills that I integrated into my training program for the next decade. I had total body awareness and I was totally prepared in any situation. Becoming a student of the sport helped me understand the sport better than many of my competitors.

## 3. Work Harder Than The Rest.

Hard work beats talent when talent doesn't work hard. To have great performances, I prepared better than anyone in the world. I had a 400m mentality (Phillips came from a 400m background), so I trained like a 400m runner and I think that really helped separate me from the rest of my competitors. I felt I could outwork anybody. I trained with all the greatest sprinters and that really helped elevate my performances. I knew I was powerful and I didn't think I could lose to anybody in the world. Where I was different is that I could do the same workouts as a 400m runner but then I would bound, lift weights and then go to the pool with an hour work out. I would do that every single day for nearly 14 years. Hard work is the foundation for every athlete – if you don't have that, you won't be successful.

# Letter to A Young Athlete

Dear Young Athlete,

Here's something I'd like to share with you that I wish someone would have told me when I was growing up and playing sport. Like it or not, you're not going to play well, or the way you'd like to, every time you step out to compete. In fact, sometimes you won't win even though you are playing your best.

The reality is you will have more days that you are not going to play or perform the way you'd like to. Part of the reason why athletes get frustrated or get down on themselves is due to their expectations. They want to play "their way" every time they step out to compete. That's impossible. Most of the time, you'll play below your expectations. Though it is a difficult reality to accept, it is the truth!

You have always got to expect the best from yourself, to be confident, and to give your very best. However, be prepared to handle the way you are going to think when you aren't playing as well as you'd like to. It will happen frequently.

You can't control the outcome of your performance, or how well you will be able to execute your techniques and tactics, even when you have properly prepared. But, you can control how you are going to react to it. Don't let negative energy rob you of your success. A bad attitude is like a flat tire, you will end up getting nowhere until you change it!

Champion minded athletes are great, not because they have brilliance, but because they are more accepting of their mistakes.

They know how to get over them and to deal with them better than other competitors. They are consistent in their routines because routines help them process mistakes while keeping a positive mindset.

That's probably the main reason they've won some of their biggest games or tournaments playing far less than their best. I once read this and it stuck, "In the heat of battle, you don't rise to your level, you sink to the habits you have created in your practices." I love this quote because it's so true. As a mindset and sports performance coach, I keep reminding the athletes I work with that you become your habits under pressure. Those habits better be good ones!

I recently read a piece on former French Open tennis champion Gaston Gaudio. This is what he said, "Most of the time you don't play the way you want, things don't go the way that you would like to, so you have to manage that."

Many years back, whilst living in South Africa, I worked with Graeme Smith, the former South African cricket captain. He commented, "I know I'm not going to play the want to every time, but I can control how I'm going to think about it."

After 8 months out with an injury, another former client of mine, 3-time World Squash Champion Ramy Ashour, went to the 2014 World Championships knowing he wasn't anywhere near 100% fit, After each match, we spoke via phone. He said, "I got through, even though not playing my best, but all that matters is that it was good enough for today to play tomorrow again." This is what a winner and a champion minded athlete understands. They accept it and they get through it!

NBA star Lebron James said, "It's impossible to play 80-odd games a season and expect to be firing on all cylinders for every game.

What matters is that I'm trying my hardest every game and putting in the work. Some players put so much pressure on themselves thinking they can rock the floor every night! It's impossible!"

In my experience working with athletes at all levels I've found that it's those with perfectionist personalities who are more likely to sabotage their own performances. They cannot accept that they aren't playing as well as they'd like to.

## 3 Realities Champion Minded Athletes Know Better Than the Rest:

1. They accept that they aren't going to play their best every time they step out to compete.

2. They understand that success lies in the consistent control of their habits, their behaviors, and their mindset.

3. They understand that in order to give themselves a chance of succeeding on their bad days, they need to continually give their best effort and believe they can actually win. They don't let a negative attitude or mindset get in the way.

The champion minded athletes understand these realities better than the rest. They know they are only as good as their bad days. But the differences is that even on their bad days, they are still able to stay positive and to perform at a high level.

So, let me ask you, *"How good are you on your bad days?"*

*Yours Sincerely,*
Coach McCaw

# It All Matters

*Champion Minded Athletes*
*Are Disciplined Even When*
*No One's Watching.*

- When you sleep in and miss a work out - it matters.

- When you skip breakfast - it matters.

- When you neglect your daily recovery routines (stretching, foam rolling, nap) - it matters.

- When you eat junk food because you didn't prepare healthy choices - it matters.

- When you cut corners during your practice or in warm ups - it matters.

- When you give less than 100% effort because coach isn't there - it matters.

- When you don't take care of your equipment - it matters.

- When you display negative body language - it matters.

- When you talk negatively to yourself - it matters.

- When you are disrespectful to parents, coaches, teammates, officials, etc. - it matters.

- When you avoid or disregard criticism and feedback - it matters.

- When you gossip about coaches, teammates, etc. - it matters.

- When you don't put your teammates first - it matters.

- When you avoid challenge and choose what is easy and familiar - it matters.

- When you don't keep notes in your journal - it matters.

- When your habits aren't in line with your goals - it matters.

- When you neglect to get enough sleep by staying out late - it matters.

- When you look to place blame instead of taking ownership - it matters.

- When you don't show gratitude and respect - it matters.

* * *

*The champion minded athlete*
*is aware that every thought and action matters.*

# Identity Crisis

*You are not defined by what you do.*

In the last few years, I've consulted with over 500 world-class athletes in a variety of sports. These elite athletes have either competed at a college, national, or international level. To reach that level, most have been wildly successful at winning. For them, winning has become an addiction.

The majority of them have been playing their chosen sport since the ages of five or six. Once they started showed signs of having some skills, they grew accustomed to being known as "Gary, the rugby player" or "Jessica, the tennis player." Throughout their playing careers, their personal identities became defined by what they did in their sports. However, after their playing careers are finished many athletes struggle to know who they really are. Up until the point of retirement, their identity was wrapped up into how they performed in the sporting arena. This is when an identity crises may occur.

When I first sit down with an athlete I ask them their life's purpose. I don't want their goals, but rather, their deeper purpose away from sport. I want to know their *why*.

All their lives what they have done has defined who they are. This can be dangerous.

You are not defined by what you do.

You are not defined by what you have achieved, won, or lost.

You are not what the newspapers, gossip magazines, or media say you are; because they don't even know you. You are who you are.

After a playing career, athletes often discover who are their real friends. Some can find it a lonely place. This is why it is so important to find your greater purpose in life. This is why it is important to find your identity in something that can never be taken away from you. This is why it's important to surround yourself with people who see you for the person you are, not for what you do or did in a sports career. Surround yourself with those who care more for you as a person than for your successes or failures on a court or field; people who accept you for your flaws and faults, people who are more interested in your future instead of your past.

\* \* \*

*It's not what you achieve that matters,*
*it's who you're becoming in pursuit of achievement.*

# Preparing for the Other 2/3

*Champion minded athletes*
*prepare for life after their sports career.*

A sports career can be very short. No matter how good you are or what titles you win, it can all end in a second. Sports careers are can be short due to injury, illness, scandal (which can lead to loss of endorsements and contracts), legal and/or financial trouble (mishandling fame and fortune). That's why, in addition to your sports skills, it's critical to work hard on your education and life skills. You need to be prepared for the next phase of life.

Tony Conigliaro, or "Tony C" as he was known by fans, had a bright future ahead of him with the Boston Red Sox. In his first three seasons, Conigliaro hit .273 with 84 home runs and 227 runs batted in. He led the league in 1965 with 32 home runs. On August 18, 1967, the Red Sox hosted the California Angels. In his third at-bat of the game, Conigliaro, who had gone two-for-two, got beaned. Back then, helmets were not what they are now. The pitch severely broke his left cheekbone, and he collapsed face first over home plate. The injury would prove to be career-ending. Though he made a valiant attempt at a comeback, his eyesight was permanently ruined. Each year, Major League Baseball gives the Tony Conigliaro Award to the player who best overcomes adversity; displaying the spirit, determination, and courage of Tony Conigliaro.

Englishman Mike Friday is one of the world's best rugby coaches. I met Mike during a training camp in San Diego, where I was consulting with the U.S. Paralympic Soccer Team. At the time, Mike was coaching the USA Rugby 7's team. A highly disciplined and driven leader, he had the following to say about life after a career in sports, "As a player, I always made sure I kept my contacts and business interests as active as possible. You always have to be prepared for that next move. I knew that rugby wouldn't last forever, so I had to make the most of every opportunity."

Retired tennis legend Andre Agassi once said, "We spend one third of our lives not really preparing for the other two thirds. After a sports career, there's a whole new other life to manage." Similarly, NFL Quarterback Peyton Manning said, "I'm totally convinced that the end of my football career is just the beginning of something I haven't even discovered yet. Life is not shrinking for me, it's morphing into a whole new world of possibilities."

\* \* \*

*The champion minded*
*are ahead of the game when it comes to*
*planning for life after sports.*

# Employers Want to Hire Former Athletes

*Champion minded athletes*
*translate the ideals of sport success to life.*

A few years back, I was chatting with one of my clients who happened to be the CEO of a successful company in Johannesburg, South Africa. In between sets, we spoke about what his company looked for when hiring new employees. Interestingly, Dane (who also happened to be a former NCAA All-American in his chosen sport) often looked to see if the job-applicant was a past athlete. They also looked to see whether the athlete excelled for their respective colleges or teams. In addition to the results and achievements of the individual, they researched how well they got along with others, how well they handled pressure, and how well they adapted to change. More importantly, they wanted to know if these individuals were team players.

## 10 reasons why athletes are great in business:

1. Athletes have a greater drive and determination to practice a task rigorously, relentlessly, and even in the midst of failure, until they succeed.

2. Athletes have a strong work ethic and the ability to deal with adversity.

3. Athletes are goal setters and love to achieve their goals.

4. Athletes are great at getting along with others since they often have better communication and social skills.

5. Athletes are able to develop new skills more easily.

6. Athletes are problem-solvers and love to strategize.

7. Athletes conserve their energy. They understand that when they take better care of their health and wellness, they will perform better.

8. Athletes are more reliable, trustworthy, and accountable.

9. Athletes are healthier, and therefore, take less sick leave days.

10. Athletes are team players.

* * *

*Always be at your best,*
*because you never know who might be watching.*

# Champion Minded For Life

*Twenty standards to enjoy success in sport and in life.*

1. Joy has little to do with your circumstances, and much to do with your focus. "Focus on the journey, not the destination. Joy is found not in finishing an activity, but in doing it." - Greg Anderson

2. Don't take yourself too seriously. "It's your outlook on life that counts. If you take yourself lightly and don't take yourself too seriously, pretty soon you can find the humor in our everyday lives. And sometimes it can be a lifesaver." - Betty White

3. Work hard. "Far and away the best prize that life has to offer is the chance to work hard at work worth doing." - Theodore Roosevelt

4. Be respectful of others even when you disagree with them. "One of the most sincere forms of respect is actually listening to what another has to say." - Bryant H. McGill

5. Be willing to do what others won't, to achieve what others thought impossible. "Today I will do what others won't, so tomorrow I can accomplish what others can't." - Jerry Rice

6. Have structure to your day with good habits and routines. "You'll never change your life until you change something you do daily. The secret of your success is found in your daily routine." - John C. Maxwell

7. Be grateful. "'Thank you' is the best prayer that anyone could say. I say that one a lot. 'Thank you' expresses extreme gratitude, humility, understanding." - Alice Walker

8. Be humble. "Being humble means recognizing that we are not on earth to see how important we can become, but to see how much difference we can make in the lives of others." - Gordon B. Hinckley

9. Be self-disciplined in your words and actions. "Self-discipline begins with the mastery of your thoughts. If you con't control what you think, you can't control what you do. Simply, self-discipline enables you to think first and act afterward." - Napoleon Hill

10. Forgive. "The weak can never forgive. Forgiveness is the attribute of the strong." - Mahatma Gandhi

11. Be positive. "Nothing can dim the light that shines from within." - Maya Angelou

12. Give others your full attention. "The most precious gift we can offer anyone is our attention. When mindfulness embraces those we love, they will bloom like flowers." - Thich Nhat Hanh

13. Be gracious in victory and graceful in defeat. "If you can meet with Triumph and Disaster and threat those two imposters just the same." - Rudyard Kipling

14. Be empathetic. Understand before you judge. "Empathy is seeing with the eyes of another, listening with the ears of another, and feeling with the heart of another." - Alfred Adler

15. Be the first to apologize. "To err is human; to forgive, divine." - Alexander Pope

16. Live simply. "Be content with what you have; rejoice in the way things are. When you realize there is nothing lacking, the whole world belongs to you." - Lao Tzu

17. Stand up straight. Make eye contact. Extend a firm handshake. "I can feel the twinkle of his eye in his handshake." - Helen Keller

18. Say 'Please' and 'Thank You'. "Politeness is a sign of dignity, not subservience." - Theodore Roosevelt

19. Be a life-long learner. "Never stop learning and adapting. The world will always be changing. If you limit yourself to what you knew and what you were comfortable with earlier in your life, you will grow increasingly frustrated with your surroundings as you age." - David Niven

20. Follow the Golden Rule. "Nothing in the Golden Rule says that others will treat us as we have treated them. If only says that we must treat others in a way that we would want to be treated." - Rosa Parks

\* \* \*

*"Mastering others is strength.*
*Mastering yourself is true power."*

- Lao Tzu

# Want to Know More?

*Invite Allistair to speak at your next event!*

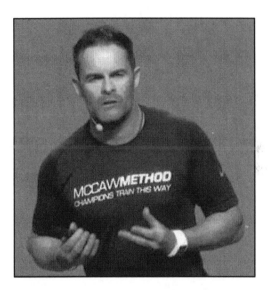

## ALLISTAIR MCCAW
### AUTHOR

Having presented in over 35 countries to National Olympic Federations, sports teams, colleges, schools, and corporations; Allistair has positively impacted the mindsets, cultures, and environments of athletes, coaches, and teams worldwide.

Regardless of the genre, when audiences seek excellence, Allistair is able to share his passion, knowledge, expertise, and vast experience working with some of the world's best performers. To enhance his presentations, he incorporates the 8 principles to becoming champion minded.

## Consulting:

- Athletes
- Coaches
- Clubs, Teams, and Colleges
- Corporations, Companies, and Organizations
- Anyone who wants to achieve greatness in his or her life!

### For more details, please contact:

*mccawmethod@gmail.com*

### You can also follow Allistair on social media:

*Twitter @allistairmccaw*

*Twitter @championminded*

*Instagram: BeChampionMinded*

*Hashtag on all social media: #ChampionMinded*

### Please visit:

*www.allistairmccaw.com*

M

**Please feel free to share your favorite quotes from this book on social media.**

**Remember to include the hashtag:**
*#ChampionMinded*

**Your feedback matters!**

*Allistair believes feedback is the key to growing and to improving. He'd love for you to take a moment and leave a short review on Amazon.com about this book!*

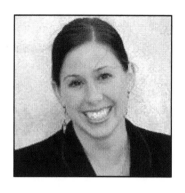

## J ENNY  W ALLS  R OBB
## C O - AUTHOR  &  E DITOR

Jenny grew up playing a variety of youth sports in Birmingham, Alabama before playing NCAA Division I tennis at Samford University, where she earned her Bachelor of Arts in English/Language Arts. Jenny is passionate about education. She is an Elite Professional in the United States Professional Tennis Association (USPTA) and earned the distinction of Master of Tennis - Junior Development, in addition to a Professional Certification in Adult Development, through the Professional Tennis Registry (PTR). Jenny is a Certified Tennis Performance Specialist with the International Tennis Performance Association (ITPA) and a faculty member of the United States Tennis Congress (USTC).

Jenny's goal as a coach is to develop athletes of good character with a solid foundation of fundamental techniques and tactics. She is passionate about promoting and growing the game of tennis at the grass roots level through her involvement in the United States Tennis Association (USTA) programs Junior Team Tennis (JTT) and National Junior Tennis and Learning (NJTL). Through her position as Director of Marketing & Communications for USTA

Alabama and USPTA Alabama President, she hopes to help raise the standards of tennis-teaching professionals and coaches.

## On social media:

*Facebook: Jenny Walls Robb*
*Twitter: @jennywrobb*
*Instagram: @jennywrobb*

# A Special Word of Thanks and Gratitude

To Craig Cignarelli, who helped put the finishing touches on this book. This project required a truly champion minded team effort from Jenny and Craig!

Thank you both so much. This would not have been possible without you.

## *Teamwork makes the dream work!*

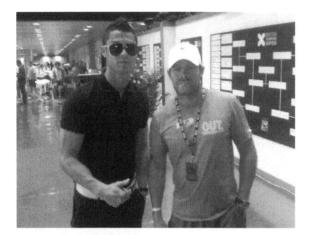

Cristiano
Ronaldo

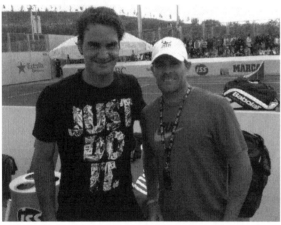

Roger
Federer

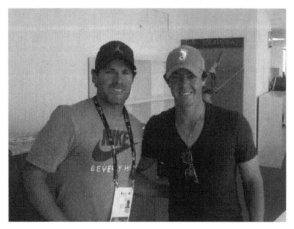

Rory
Mcilroy

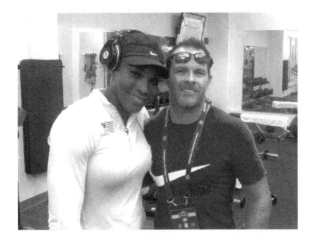

Serena
Williams

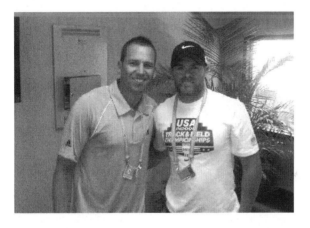

Sergio
Garcia

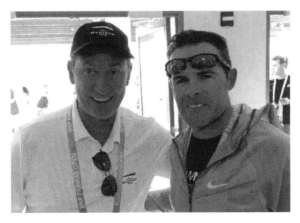

Wayne
Gretzky

# Notes

Printed in Great Britain
by Amazon